THE LITTLE BOOK OF
ENERGY HEALING TECHNIQUES

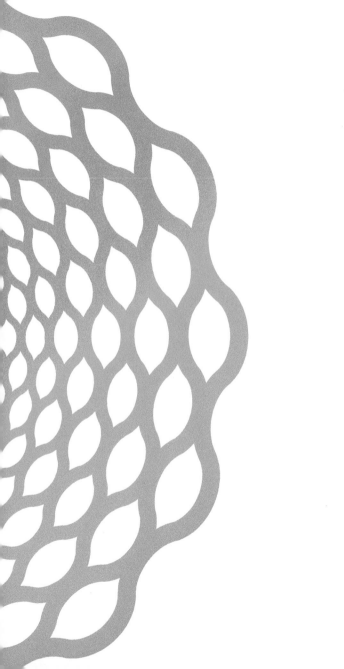

The Little Book of

ENERGY HEALING

TECHNIQUES

Simple Practices to Heal
Body, Mind, and Spirit

KAREN FRAZIER

ALTHEA
PRESS

For general information on our other products and services or to obtain technical support, please contact our Customer Care Department within the United States at (866) 744-2665, or outside the United States at (510) 253-0500.

Althea Press publishes its books in a variety of electronic and print formats. Some content that appears in print may not be available in electronic books, and vice versa.

TRADEMARKS: Althea Press and the Althea Press logo are trademarks or registered trademarks of Callisto Media Inc. and/or its affiliates, in the United States and other countries, and may not be used without written permission. All other trademarks are the property of their respective owners. Althea Press is not associated with any product or vendor mentioned in this book.

Interior and Cover Designer: Will Mack
Art Producer: Sue Smith
Editor: Stacy Wagner-Kinnear
Production Manager: Kim Ciabattari
Production Editor: Melissa Edeburn

Illustration: © 2019 Conor Buckley, pp. 8, 23,24,25, 26, 27, 51, 98, 115, 135, 142, and 144; all other interior Illustrations © Shutterstock.

Photography: © Shutterstock, pp. 55, 57, 62, 63, 64, and 65; © iStock, p. 62 (black tourmaline); © Lucia Loisa, p. 63 (rose quartz).

Author photo: Courtesy ©Tristan David Luciotti.

ISBN: Print 978-1-64152-548-0 | eBook 978-1-64152-549-7

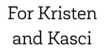

For Kristen
and Kasci

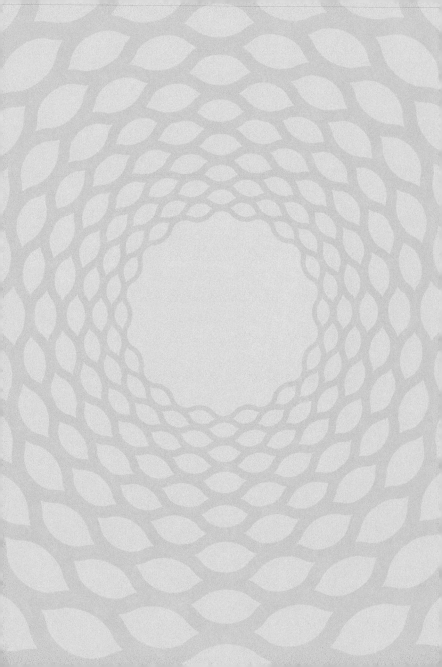

CONTENTS

THE ENERGY HEALING JOURNEY

Energy healing plays an important role in my life. I've been writing and blogging about it for more than a decade, and it's a practice that I not only teach but also *live* every day.

Although I've only dedicated the past 10 or so years to sharing energy healing with others, my own energy healing journey began in 1991, when I went to work for a chiropractor. I was in my late twenties and already had an avid interest in alternative and natural healing techniques because traditional Western medicine was unable to help me overcome my chronic health issues. In my new job, I learned a different way to view health: from the perspective of body, mind, and spirit balance. The experience changed my understanding of what health is and how I could attain and maintain it. The nearly 10 years I spent working there provided the foundational knowledge that I used as a springboard to become an energy healer.

There is a saying in chiropractic, attributed to its founder, B. J. Palmer: "The power that made the body heals the body." The first time I heard this insight, it resonated deeply. It was at the forefront of my mind as I began to take a new approach to my health whenever I struggled with an acute condition that wouldn't go away.

I'd been suffering from a severe sore throat for weeks, and conventional medicine, homeopathy, naturopathy, and chiropractic adjustments weren't helping. In desperation, I sought care from a medical doctor/energy healer who worked with various modalities—none that I'd ever heard of or necessarily believed in, but I figured I'd take my chances. At my appointment, the doctor used crystals and hands-on healing, and I felt a physical and emotional rush as something released inside me, and my sore throat was gone instantly. I felt fantastic. It was then that I truly understood the power of energy healing, so I began to learn about it in earnest.

I started with crystals and essential oils, learning how I could use them to make changes in my body, mind, and spirit. From there, I journeyed into Eastern philosophy, meditation, affirmation, visualization, and Reiki. And then my interest snowballed. I've spent the past 20 years learning everything I could about various forms of energy healing by becoming a Reiki Master/ Teacher, mastering and practicing other energy healing modalities, and earning bachelor's, master's, and PhD degrees in metaphysical science. In the past few years, I've incorporated an old love (music) into my energy healing practices as well. I'm learning sound energetics from a master of Tibetan sound healing and pursuing a DD (doctor of divinity) degree in spiritual healing with an emphasis on how sound affects vibration.

This is my sixth book about energy healing. I teach energy healing classes and offer healing sound bath meditations throughout the Pacific Northwest because

I'm passionate about empowering others to heal using vibrational techniques. I practice Reiki, crystal healing, sound healing, and other energy healing modalities with clients, friends, family, animals, and—perhaps most important—myself.

Your body, mind, and spirit have innate intelligence. There is a creative force—call it God, the Divine, Universal Intelligence, Source Energy, or whatever fits your belief system—that created you and continues to operate intelligently within you. Energy healing reconnects you with this intelligence, helping the power that made your body heal it. Even simple techniques used for a few minutes a day, a few times a week, can set you on the journey to emotional, spiritual, mental, and physical well-being.

What This Book Is

This book provides simple, practical vibrational healing techniques to balance the energy of your body, mind, and spirit. The following are some of the specific individual practices and techniques you will learn:

- Healing mindset
- Intention
- Meditation
- Hands-on healing
- Sound healing
- Crystals
- Aromatherapy

You can use any of these techniques to begin creating energetic shifts that allow your innate intelligence to balance your energy to spark healing. When you establish daily practices that incorporate these tools, your energy can begin to shift in various aspects of your life.

This book is a step along your journey toward self-healing; one that will encourage you to seek a new understanding of what healing is and how you can start to change your life.

What This Book Is Not

This book doesn't guarantee you'll never experience "dis-ease" (lack of ease of the body, mind, and spirit) again. Nor is it intended to magically make everything in your life perfect. Energy healing is a process that helps you create energetic balance, but it doesn't necessarily offer an instant cure. In fact, vibrational imbalances that manifest as dis-ease often exist to help you discover something important. Sometimes this learning process requires more than a single healing session or technique to overcome the symptoms dis-ease creates.

Likewise, this book won't train you to work with clients. It is not intended as a comprehensive book of energy healing techniques; nor is it a substitute for training with a qualified professional to start a practice. It's also not meant to be the only energy healing book you ever purchase. You won't find the following advanced techniques covered in this book:

- Reiki
- Acupuncture/ acupressure
- Traditional Chinese medicine
- Homeopathy
- Hypnotherapy
- Ayurveda

However, if you are trained in these or other modalities and feel they may be helpful to you, you can substitute them for other techniques, such as touch. With the recommended techniques, always rely on your best instincts to personalize your experience in energy healing.

1
~

An Introduction to Energy Healing

Energy healing has been a powerful force in my life, and I've seen it work wonders for others as well. Some have experienced a series of small shifts that led to better states of overall well-being; others have seen significant change, such as a cessation of symptoms or a shift in their overall health. Some have even been cured of specific conditions. What I've discovered with energy healing is that it works differently for everyone, bringing about shifts of body, mind, spirit, and awareness that serve the highest and greatest good of everyone involved.

What Is Healing?

Healing means different things to different people. For some, it may mean no more symptoms. To others, it may mean remission or absence of dis-ease (energetic imbalances of body, mind, or spirit). Ideas about healing might include the following:

- Disappearance or absence of symptoms

- Remission or absence of physical illness

- Achieving optimal physical, emotional, spiritual, or mental health

- Balance of body, mind, and spirit

- Removal of blockages that cause imbalance

In other words, your definition of healing is probably different from anyone else's because your personal wellness picture is uniquely yours. Likewise, your definition of healing may be a moving target throughout your life. For our purposes, I'll define healing in a way that meets this moving target. *Healing* is creating shifts that bring about positive changes in wellness that serve the highest and greatest good.

What Is Energy Healing?

Energy healing is a broad term describing techniques and practices that change the energetic vibration of something to facilitate balance. Each of these techniques affects life force energy—sometimes called *prana* or *chi*—by removing blockages and balancing excessive vibration to create unobstructed, balanced energy flow. We use energy healing to remove dis-ease by correcting imbalances in our physical (body and mind) or etheric (emotions and spirit) energies.

Energy healing has been practiced for thousands of years. Here are a few examples:

- Ancient Chinese energy healing beliefs and prac- tices date back more than 6,000 years and include the concept of chi; the energetic balance of the five elements—metal, wood, fire, water, and earth: the idea of energetic meridians, or channels, used in acupuncture; and the balance of yin and yang.

- Ayurveda, the traditional Hindu system of medi- cine, and its concepts of balancing the three doshas (pitta, kapha, and vata) and five elements (ether, air, fire, water, and earth) also extend back over 6,000 years, in India.

- Yoga, with its focus on the intentional movement of prana, originated in India around 3000 BCE.

- Some believe that the miracles attributed to Jesus more than 2,000 years ago occurred because he used a form of energy healing and stated that others could carry out the same healing work (John 14:12).

All these ancient energy healing arts continue to be practiced today, and new ones have sprung up with similar traditions and their own guiding philosophies and techniques.

Unfortunately, many dismiss energy healing because it differs from the practice of Western medicine, which focuses on the physical realm: It treats your body and mind (the physical) but fails to treat your etheric (emotional and spiritual) self. Western medicine diagnoses and treats you as a series of malfunctioning biological parts. When you experience symptoms, you receive physical treatment or take medication. In this model, you are minimally active in your care.

Conversely, energy healing treats you as an interdependent energetic system comprising the physical (body and mind) and the etheric (emotions and spirit). It seeks to balance physical and etheric energy so you can achieve a higher vibrational state, expressed as better overall health.

When dis-ease occurs, the energy healer seeks to correct imbalances. In this process, you are essential to your own care. Healers facilitate or channel healing energy, but it's ultimately up to you to engage meaningfully in the energy balancing practices. As a result, when I work with people in my energy healing practices, I prefer to call them "healing partners." Your role in your healing is far more important than mine ever will be. Without your willing intention to engage in the process of healing, it is unlikely you'll improve.

Energy Healing Applications

Energy healing can have an impact that extends beyond you. As I'll explain later in this chapter, when two objects vibrating at different frequencies are in proximity, they move toward a middle vibrational point, where they lock into phase and vibrate at a new frequency. In other words, your vibrational frequency has the potential to raise or lower the frequency of other living beings, objects, and places when you are nearby, because their energy and yours will move to meet somewhere in the middle.

With this in mind, there are a number of potential applications for energy healing:

- Changing your own life or circumstances

- Empowering others to change their lives or circumstances

- Bringing vibrational shifts to spaces where you live, work, and play

- Positively affecting vibration and facilitating healing after a natural disaster or tragic event

- Helping change the planet's vibration to bring about family, societal, or worldwide healing

- Helping raise the vibration of the universe in order for the universe to evolve

In other words, you are very important. Your energy affects the energy of the whole, and by raising your vibration, you can facilitate growth and change not only for your own purposes, but also for the universe as a whole.

ENERGY HEALING IN THIS BOOK

For our purposes, when discussing energy healing, I am talking about any activity you engage in that will shift your vibrational frequency. As I previously mentioned, healing doesn't necessarily mean getting rid of illness; instead, it refers to making vibrational shifts in your own energetic systems to create balance and harmony, remove blockages, reduce overactive energy, and increase underactive vibration. I use the terms *vibration* and *energy* interchangeably; all energy is vibration, and every part of you, physical or etheric, is made up of oscillating strands of energy (envision the swinging motion of a pendulum). Therefore, when you change and balance vibration, you create a shift that helps your entire being experience more harmony and balance. These shifts always serve your highest and greatest good.

As we move forward, I will discuss various modalities that can help create this energetic balance, from hands-on techniques like tapping or simple touch, to using sound as a vibrational tool, to using other items that have a higher vibration, such as essential oils and crystals. Likewise, activities like affirmation, meditation, and visualization are healing tools that change your vibrational state by helping you overcome the persistent thoughts arising from programming and unrecognized beliefs that keep you from healing.

Vibration

Vibration is the movement of energy. Everything in the universe consists of energy vibrating at different frequencies (speeds), including how life force energy oscillates in different parts of your etheric and physical bodies. In sound, the frequency of the vibration determines the tone you hear. In vision, the frequency of the vibration is the color you perceive the object to be.

When your energy isn't balanced, the part of your physical or etheric body where the imbalance exists is not vibrating at an optimal frequency. Different energy healing techniques help move your vibration to the desirable frequency through entrainment (see page 10) to create harmony or balance that expresses as health.

HOW TO SENSE VIBRATION

Here is a simple exercise you can try to begin perceiving vibration:

1. Vigorously rub your hands together for 30 seconds to one minute.

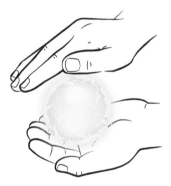

2. With your hands slightly cupped, palms facing each other, slowly pull your hands apart, noticing the tingling between them. This is vibration.

3. Continue to pull your hands apart until the tingling lessens or stops. Then, move your hands slowly back toward each other, feeling where you can start to sense the vibration again and when it stops.

You can also sense vibration through sound. Close your eyes and hum for 30 seconds or so. As you do, notice how and where you feel the vibration in your body.

COMPLEMENTARY MEDICINE, NOT ALTERNATIVE MEDICINE

Energy healing isn't an alternative to proper medical care; nor does it work at cross-purposes with your medical care. Rather, it allows you to be an active partner in your own healing. For example, if you have a wound that requires stitches, seek appropriate medical treatment first. If your appendix bursts, you need surgery. Then, once you're on the road to recovery, use energy healing as complementary care to help your body, mind, and spirit heal.

Be sure to continue medical treatment while you focus your energy healing efforts on uncovering vibrational causes. For example, I continue to take thyroid medication for Hashimoto's thyroiditis because blood tests show I need medicine. This situation may change as I continue to work on healing the vibrational issues that underlie the condition, but, for now, medical treatment is the best way to support my health. With vibrational healing, however, I've noticed many of the symptoms that used to bother me, even while on medication, have lessened or gone away.

CONTINUED

Mainstream medical studies are beginning to show that complementary forms of healing can supplement patient care. Here are just a few examples: A study reported in *Journal of Affective Disorders* shows that acupuncture was effective in treating depression, and as reported in *HealthCMI*, studies show acupuncture, particularly, can help reduce depression after a stroke. Studies published in *Translational Neurodegeneration* reveal that acupuncture and traditional Chinese medicine are effective in helping with memory in Alzheimer's patients.

ENTRAINMENT

In energy healing, when we use an object such as a singing bowl, an essential oil, or a crystal, we are using *entrainment* to bring our vibration into alignment with the vibration of the object. Dutch scientist Christiaan Huygens discovered entrainment in the 1600s when he hung two pendulum clocks near one another that were moving at different frequencies. After a short time, the pendulums began to sway together. This experiment is repeatable. You can find videos of multiple mechanical objects locking into phase in this way on my website, AuthorKarenFrazier.com.

Entrainment is how energy healing works. When you place an object vibrating at one frequency near an object vibrating at a different frequency, they lock into phase: one vibrates higher, and the other vibrates lower. It's why, in this book, you'll be working with high-vibration objects and thoughts—so that as you do, your energy will meet the thought or object's energy in the middle.

When Energy Is Unbalanced or Blocked

Energy can become overactive, underactive, or completely blocked for many reasons, such as illness, injury, negative thoughts, subconscious projections, unrecognized beliefs, childhood issues or trauma, misunderstandings, relationship problems, past-life trauma, chemical toxicity, poor nutrition, lack of movement, emotional pain, spiritual confusion, and many other issues. In fact, virtually any negative experience in your physical or etheric body can cause energy to become unbalanced or even blocked. The longer you go without correcting or removing what is causing the imbalance, the more out of balance your energies become.

Eastern philosophies teach that energy needs to be balanced between polar opposites, such as yin and yang, dark and light, or feminine and masculine, as well as among the five elemental energies: earth, metal, wood, water, and air. In other philosophies, such as Ayurveda, you may see these elements called something slightly different, such as fire, water, earth, air, and ether (or aether). Everything, including your physical and etheric bodies, optimally contains a balance of both polar energies and elemental energies. When these energies are out of balance, the result is dis-ease.

SYMPTOMS

As I mentioned, dis-ease is different from disease or illness. Dis-ease is a state of imbalance. It causes your higher guidance (which I call the Divine guidance system) to send symptoms to indicate something is not balanced.

Symptoms may be physical, emotional, mental, circumstantial, or spiritual. Initially, symptoms are usually something simple and relatively minor, such as a mild headache, a disturbing dream, or a vague feeling of discomfort or sadness. However, as the imbalance becomes more serious, symptoms grow stronger and louder. When an imbalance has gone unaddressed for a long period and becomes severe, your Divine guidance system may send extreme symptoms, which I call the "universal two-by-four" (the universe smacks you upside the head with a two-by-four so that you pay attention). Examples of these symptoms include a heart attack, a job loss, a major depression, or a "dark night of the soul." Typically, the more severe your symptoms, the more serious the imbalance is and the sooner you need to correct it.

In Western society, we often react to symptoms by either ignoring them or doing something (such as taking medication) to remove or suppress them. However, symptoms are like your Divine guidance system's smoke detector. Treating the symptoms without trying to find the cause is akin to removing the batteries from your smoke detector to stop it from beeping, instead of trying to discover and remove the cause of the smoke. Eventually the whole building is going to burn to the ground.

The longer we ignore or suppress the symptoms, the more ingrained the imbalance becomes and the more effort it takes to remove it. However, no symptom is ever so severe that we lose the ability to rebalance our energy and start to heal our body, mind, and spirit.

Often, we assume we know what a symptom means because of where or how it occurs. But sometimes a symptom and cause appear unrelated. If foot pain occurs due to a blockage of the sciatic nerve, treating the foot would be pointless because the imbalance is elsewhere in the body. Once you begin to recognize how the body, mind, and spirit work together through the energy body and its various parts, you can begin to trace symptoms to their root, where the imbalance exists.

Remember: We aren't a series of disparate parts. We exist holistically, as body, mind, and spirit.

CHAKRAS

- ● CROWN CHAKRA
- ● THIRD EYE CHAKRA
- ● THROAT CHAKRA
- ● HEART CHAKRA
- ● SOLAR PLEXUS CHAKRA
- ● SACRAL CHAKRA
- ● ROOT CHAKRA

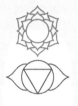

The Energy Body

You are pure energy. Some of that energy manifests as your physical body, and some manifests as your spiritual or etheric body. Physically manifested beings (which is what we are when we inhabit a human body) have specific energy systems that connect the physical to the etheric. Within these systems, you can create balance and harmony to bring about healing. And although you don't need to be an energy body scholar to begin the process of your own energy healing, getting familiar with the basics of these systems is helpful. I will teach you when and how to work with each system in the daily routines in chapter 3 and the condition-specific remedies in chapter 4.

CHAKRAS

I love working with chakras because they are one of the easiest energy systems to identify and visualize. Chakras are whirling wheels of energy that run roughly along your spinal column and connect your physical body to your etheric body. Each of the chakras has a different vibrational frequency that corresponds to different colors and tones (sounds). Likewise, your chakras correspond to different physical aspects of your body (those areas roughly located near or just downstream or upstream from each chakra), and imbalances in certain chakras can create physical, mental, emotional, spiritual, or situational dis-ease.

The word chakra comes from the Sanskrit cakra, which means "wheel." Chakras were first described in the Vedas, ancient Hindu scriptures written in Sanskrit that date somewhere between 1500 BCE and 500 BCE. Similar concepts of energy centers are also discussed in various other traditions, including Jewish mysticism (Kabbalah) and Buddhism.

Imbalances in the chakras tend to arise from over-active energy, underactive energy, or blocked energy. When energy doesn't flow unhindered, in a balanced fashion, the result is dis-ease in the physical and etheric areas that correspond with the chakras.

The various energy healing tools discussed in the next chapter can help rebalance energy so it flows freely through the chakras, restoring your life force and removing dis-ease from your physical and etheric bodies. A guide to energy healing tools that work well with each chakra is included near the end of the book (see page 150), so you can use it as a quick reference for rebalancing.

ROOT CHAKRA

The root chakra is the first chakra, some-times called the base chakra or Muladhara. It is located at the base of your spine. It vibrates in the color red and is associated with the physical areas of the body, including your lower extremities and the base of your spine.

Physical issues associated with the root chakra include leg and foot issues, sciatica, lower back pain, immune system problems, and hemorrhoids. Emotional and spiritual issues with root chakra imbalance might include identity problems, safety and security issues, the inability to stand up for yourself, depression, and fear of abandonment.

SACRAL CHAKRA

The sacral chakra is the second chakra, sometimes called the spleen chakra or Svadisthana. It vibrates in the color orange and is located a few inches below your navel.

Physical issues associated with the sacral chakra include problems with the sexual organs, intestines, and pelvic region. Emotional and spiritual issues associated with this chakra include an inability to form creative ideas, issues related to sexuality, difficulty with prosperity, and issues of control and personal power.

SOLAR PLEXUS CHAKRA

The third chakra, the solar plexus chakra, is also called the navel chakra or Manipura. It is located a few inches below the small extension of bone just below your rib cage (or xiphoid process) in your solar plexus region. It vibrates in the color yellow. You will also find the color gold associated with this chakra.

Physically, your solar plexus chakra affects your stomach, liver, spleen, kidneys, and gallbladder as well as your lower mid-back region. Physical issues arising from imbalance might include diabetes, adrenal exhaustion, kidney stones, ulcers, and acid reflux, whereas emotional and spiritual issues might include exhaustion, poor self-esteem, narcissism and egotism, other personality issues, social awkwardness, and eating disorders.

HEART CHAKRA

The fourth chakra is the heart chakra, also called Anahata. In the heart chakra, your energy transitions from dense and primarily physical to etheric and emotional. It is located in the center of your chest and vibrates in the color green; you will also find the color pink associated with this chakra.

Physical areas associated with the heart chakra include the heart, lungs, circulatory system, and upper thoracic region. Physical issues arising from imbalance might include lung and heart disease, blood vessel disease and circulation problems, and breast issues. Emotional and spiritual issues associated with imbalance include the inability to forgive, stuck grief, anger, bitterness, and loneliness.

THROAT CHAKRA

The fifth chakra is the throat chakra. It is also called Vishuddha. It is located just above your thyroid gland in the center of your throat, and it vibrates in the color blue.

Physically, the throat chakra affects the areas of the throat, upper chest, mouth, esophagus, gums, teeth, and ears. Physical issues associated with throat chakra imbalance include thyroid problems, gum disease, dental problems, and temporomandibular joint disorder (TMJ). Mental, emotional, and spiritual issues might include judgment and criticism, the inability to speak one's truth, poor self-expression, an unwillingness to surrender personal will to Divine will, and poor decision-making skills.

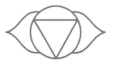

THIRD EYE CHAKRA

The third eye chakra is the sixth chakra, and it's also known as the pineal chakra or Ajna. It's located in the center of your forehead. This chakra vibrates in the color purple or violet.

Third eye chakra imbalances might physically manifest as headaches, sinus or eye problems, or poor sleep. Mental and emotional issues associated with imbalances may include a lack of critical thinking, poor reasoning skills, closed-mindedness, or low emotional intelligence.

CROWN CHAKRA

The crown chakra, also called Sahasrara, is the seventh chakra. It is located at the top of your head. It vibrates in the color white.

Imbalances in the crown chakra might cause physical issues such as systemic health problems, bone problems, skin disorders, and various mental health imbalances. Emotional and spiritual issues associated with imbalance might include a poor sense of ethics, lack of trust, and lack of belief in anything greater than oneself.

AURAS

The word aura means "wind" or "breath." It describes the energy field that surrounds you and emanates from you (and other objects and beings). According to the *Dictionary of Gnosis and Western Esotericism*, the idea of auras actually originated during the Spiritualist era of the late 1800s in the Theosophical Society, which proposed that bands of energy surround living beings in layers of bright colors that roughly correspond to chakra colors. Aura colors can change day to day or minute to minute as they reflect your current state of physical, emotional, mental, and spiritual well-being. Some psychics are able to see auras and aura colors, and aura photographs use biodynamic feedback and LED lights to visualize how colors might look surrounding the subject.

We won't do much work with auras in this book, although I can offer a quick energy technique to sweep your aura if you're feeling "off." While you sit or stand, have someone place their hands at the crown of your head, but a few inches above the surface of your skin. Starting there, have them run their hands all the way down to your feet. They should sweep on all sides of the body, flicking any energy from their fingers into the earth and ending with touching the floor, to ground you and them and disconnect your energy from theirs.

ELEMENTAL ENERGIES

All matter consists of different types of elemental energies. There are five elemental energies that need to be in balance within organisms or spaces in order to create harmony, balance, and well-being. Polarity therapy, a hands-on wellness practice to balance energies, focuses on the four classical elements (earth, water, air, and fire) proposed in ancient Greece, along with a fifth element, ether, which was added later by Aristotle. These five elements also roughly correspond to the five elements (wood, fire, earth, metal, and water) in Taoism, a Chinese philosophy.

Like the chakras, each element is associated with certain physical, spiritual, and emotional characteristics. The elemental energies flow through channels in your body from your toes and fingers to the top of your head, as illustrated in the accompanying diagrams.

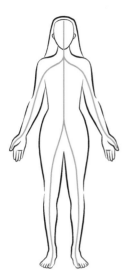

ETHER

Meaning: Space

Chakra association: Throat

Fingers and toes: Thumbs, big toes

Organ association: Ears

Characteristics: Spirituality and airiness; ether is the most subtle of the elements and is present in all four of the other elements

Location: Center of the head down the midline of the body, connecting with the thumbs, midline, and big toes

Too much ether: Ungrounded, flighty, empty-headed, vacant or vapid, dormant, and awaiting an outside force to cause movement and growth

Too little ether: May lack the room to grow or change; may be stuck in his or her ways; may have very heavy, slow-moving energy

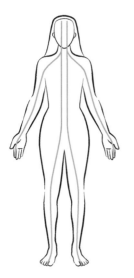

AIR

Meaning: Liveliness, lightness, and movement

Chakra association: Heart

Fingers and toes: Index fingers, second toes

Organ association: Heart

Characteristics: Movement, airiness, flow, the ability to shift quickly

Location: Moves in two channels down the body a few inches on either side of the midline, through the brows, along the outer curve of the lips, next to the chin, downward along either side of the navel, and into the index fingers and second toes of each hand and foot

Too much air: May lack boundaries and follow wherever they are led; might be considered an "airhead" due to frequently misplacing items or forgetting what they're saying while speaking; may also be prone to nervousness, anxiety, or obsessions and compulsions

Too little air: May be inflexible, overly critical, or stuck in their ways; may feel "heavy" or listless; may feel joyless or humorless

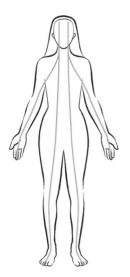

FIRE

Meaning: Bright, hot, passionate, and vivid

Chakra association: Solar plexus

Fingers and toes: Middle

Organ association: Digestive organs

Characteristics: Hot, bile, passion, active, fast moving, bright, driven

Location: A few inches out from the air channels on either side, running down the cheeks, across the nipples, along the rib cage, and down through the middle fingers of each hand and the middle toes of each foot

Too much fire: May experience restlessness, sleeplessness, fever, sexual compulsion, stress, lack of concern about others' boundaries, and burning out

Too little fire: May experience joylessness and lack of passion or drive

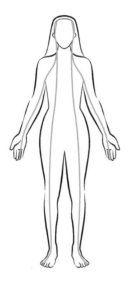

WATER

Meaning: Emotions

Chakra association: Sacral

Fingers and toes: Ring fingers, fourth toes

Organ association: Genitals

Characteristics: Receptive but active; flows easily, moving around obstacles or moving them aside

Location: A few inches outside of either of the fire channels, moving down along the sides of the head, the ears, and the outer chest, and flowing downward through the ring fingers and fourth toes of each hand and foot

Too much water: May be overly emotional or too flexible; moods and emotions may be easily affected by those around them; may have a certain formlessness to their personality and desires

Too little water: May be inflexible and emotionally dry; may be out of touch with their emotional and spiritual needs

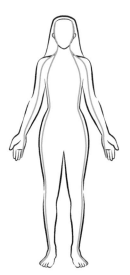

EARTH

Meaning: Grounded and stable energy

Chakra association: Root

Fingers and toes: Pinkies and little toes

Organ association: Rectum, colon

Characteristics: Heaviest of the elements, difficult to move, grounded; often moves only slowly and sluggishly; nourishes, balances

Location: Moves down through the shoulders, a few inches away from the edges of the body on either side, and down through the pinkies and little toes

Too much earth: May be slow moving, stubborn, and obstinate; may be extremely resistant to change or slow to change; may move slowly and be slow in thoughts, words, and actions; may see the world in black and white

Too little earth: May lack groundedness and centeredness; may often seem as if they are going to float away; may think or speak so quickly that they can't keep up with their own thoughts and words

POLES

Energy is also balanced among polar opposites, which are also complementary. In Taoist philosophy, which originated in ancient China circa 500 BCE, these two poles are referred to as yin and yang. One cannot exist without the other. There must be a balance of these polar energies to create harmony and ease.

YIN

Yin represents the earth and the moon. It is dark energy that is feminine in nature. Yin governs matter. It represents creative potential, contraction, and dormancy. It is internally focused, receptive, quiet, deep, and still. Yin energy is in the interior of the body (organs, veins, muscles), and it governs bodily fluids and blood.

YANG

Yang represents the sun and the heavens. It is light, bright, and masculine. Yang governs energy. It is active, aggressive, vital, externally focused, and expanding. Yang represents ambition. It governs the cycles of growth and expansion, as well as the exterior of the body and its life force energy.

MERIDIANS

Acupuncture/acupressure and traditional Chinese medicine work with energy, or chi, which, like nerves, flows in channels, or meridians, throughout your body. However, these channels are energetic and connect the physical to the etheric, whereas nerves are strictly physical. When chi is obstructed, it creates dis-ease. Acupuncture, acupressure, tapping, and various other modalities seek to remove blockages from the meridians to return the flow of chi to its optimal balanced state.

There are 12 standard meridian pathways divided into yin and yang, energies that are polar opposites but need to be balanced in order to create optimal well-being. There are six yin meridians and six yang meridians. Each corresponds to various issues and qualities. Refer to the accompanying diagram to see the correspondence of each of the meridians to the physical body.

The yin meridians include the following:

Lung (Arm Tai Yin)—acceptance, communication, grief, justice, release, receptiveness

Spleen (Leg Tai Yin)—prosperity, integrity, self-esteem, the subconscious, anxiety, the ability to receive, purification, cleansing

Heart (Arm Shao Yin)—love, acceptance, harmony and balance, peace, forgiveness, sadness, joy

YIN MERIDIANS

- LUNG (ARM TAI YIN)
- SPLEEN (LEG TAI YIN)
- HEART (ARM SHAO YIN)
- KIDNEY (LEG SHAO YIN)
- PERICARDIUM (ARM JUE YIN)
- LIVER (LEG JUE YIN)

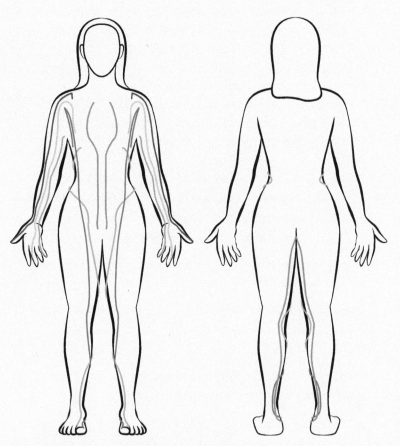

YANG MERIDIANS

- LARGE INTESTINE (ARM YANG MING)
- STOMACH (LEG YANG MING)
- SMALL INTESTINE (ARM TAI YANG)
- BLADDER (LEG TAI YANG)
- TRIPLE BURNER (ARM SHAO YANG)
- GALLBLADDER (LEG SHAO YANG)

Kidney (Leg Shao Yin)—courage, belonging, drive, paranoia, clarity, wisdom, caution, vitality, self-worth

Pericardium (Arm Jue Yin)—self-love, self-protectiveness, openness, vulnerability, self-expression

Liver (Leg Jue Yin)—benevolence, kindness, faith, destiny, hope, anger, resentment, vision, strength

The yang meridians include the following:

Large Intestine (Arm Yang Ming)—confusion, grief, control, stubbornness, regret, compulsion

Stomach (Leg Yang Ming)—criticism, gullibility, strength, grounding, intolerance, rejection, food issues, nourishment (physical and spiritual)

Small Intestine (Arm Tai Yang)—discernment, confidence, knowledge, self-destruction, intellect

Bladder (Leg Tai Yang)—anger, rage, suspicion, bitterness, jealousy, enthusiasm, intimacy, hedonism, sexuality, willpower, resentment

Triple Burner (Arm Shao Yang)—the fight-flight-freeze response, boundaries, guilt, friendship, coordination

Gallbladder (Leg Shao Yang)—assertiveness, release, anger, movement, motivation, flexibility

HOW TO HEAL

Here are some basic practices to help you develop more clarity and live more intentionally:

Identify your issues. The first step is to identify the dis-ease. See if you can identify the source of the imbalance based on what you learned in this chapter.

Practice self-honesty without judgment. As you examine your issues, be honest with yourself, which is difficult to do without self-judgment. But try to step back; notice how you feel, how past issues affect you, and how your behaviors may affect these issues.

Assess whether you're ready to let go. Ask, "Am I ready to release this issue, or is it still serving me in some way?" If you feel the issue still serves you, examine how and why. Is this choice in your best interest, or does it hold you back?

Set your intention to heal. Because intention is everything, intending to heal is the most power-ful step. Do this step silently, aloud, in writing, in meditation, or whenever it feels most appropri-ate to you.

CONTINUED

Use your tools. The upcoming chapters will provide you with tools to heal energetic imbalances. For general wellness, use the daily routines in chapter 3. For specific healing, use the tools in chapter 2 and the remedies in chapter 4.

Continue emotional and spiritual work.
Maintaining balance is an ongoing process that requires commitment, so continue your emotional and spiritual work as long as you need to.

Express gratitude. Even if your issue is still present, express gratitude for the healing process. Thank your Divine guidance system for the warnings, and thank yourself for doing the work.

Celebrate self-care. Healing requires focus, honesty, self-compassion, and dedication. Celebrate your self-love, and offer gratitude to every aspect of yourself—body, mind, and spirit—for embarking on the process of deep self-healing.

I don't work with meridians a lot, but they play an important role in your energy systems. The primary tools I've included for working with meridians are tapping and touch, which can help remove blockages or an imbalance that leads to dis-ease so the energy can flow freely once again.

Next Steps

This book offers you an introduction to energy healing, but its primary purpose in the following chapters is to offer you practical tools you can use to balance energy, cure dis-ease, and begin to heal. I also offer specific routines and processes that you can adapt to meet your own needs. Use tools that resonate with you. If you feel uncomfortable with any of the tools I suggest, feel free to adapt them in a way that feels right to you.

In the next chapter, you'll find an energy healing toolkit with an array of basic tools you can use in your energy healing practices. I offer daily routines, but your intuition plays a role here, too. If you are drawn to a specific tool for a certain situation, give it a try. Your Divine guidance system is here to help you as you start your healing journey.

Having a daily routine gets you in the mindset for healing. This book provides two daily routines you can use as a regular practice. One takes 5 minutes, and the other takes 15 minutes. Choose one or the other on the basis of your level of comfort and the time that's available to you. You can choose to perform one of these routines once or twice a day, or you can go straight to the energy healing remedies in chapter 4 and work with specific techniques to address issues you've identified.

You can also incorporate any of the tools in the following chapter or remedies in chapter 4 into your daily routine, or you can use them at a different time of day, depending on how you're feeling and how much time you have. I perform my daily practice first thing in the morning and right before going to bed, and each lasts 15 to 30 minutes. If you only have 5 minutes a day, choose one tool, one remedy, or the 5-minute routine. In the end, it doesn't matter where you start. What matters is your genuine intent to heal.

2

Your Energy Healing Toolkit

By now, you may realize you don't need to be an energy healer to facilitate vibrational healing in your own life. You can use a number of simple tools to begin to create energetic shifts in your life that will balance your physical and etheric energy to bring about changes in body, mind, and spirit that serve your highest and greatest good. Your intentional and consistent use of the seven main tools outlined in this chapter can help you begin to clear blockages and create balance and harmony in aspects of your life and being.

The Healing Mindset

Your mind plays a powerful role in bringing about healing through energy balancing. To have the best chance to facilitate healing, you'll need these skills:

Focus. It's essential to maintain focus on your goal to heal.

Positive emotion. Positive emotions have a higher vibration than negative emotions, so intentionally cultivating qualities such as gratitude, joy, and peace can help bring about positive energetic change.

Discipline. For your healing tools and practices to become a habit, you need the discipline to engage in them daily for about 10 weeks. Habitual use of your tools exponentially increases your chance of healing.

Flexibility. Frequently during the healing process, you'll discover emotions and beliefs that cause energetic blockages that have hung around for decades. To truly heal, you need the flexibility to delve into these issues as they arise and heal them before returning to your original goal.

Maintaining a healing mindset can help keep you from slipping backward into negativity, unproductive habits, and rigid thinking, which can delay or derail the healing process.

BLAME VERSUS RESPONSIBILITY

When I teach energy healing classes, inevitably someone asks a variation of this question: "Are you saying I'm to blame for my illness?" I dislike the word *blame*. It's judgmental and implies we are consciously creating illness due to some defect of strength or character. This simply isn't the case.

Yes, I believe that everyone is responsible for everything that occurs in their life, but this doesn't mean they are to blame for it. Each of us does the best we can in any given moment with the tools we have available. In the case of energetic imbalances, we often aren't aware they exist. But just because we didn't consciously create the imbalance doesn't mean we aren't responsible for it.

Everything that arises, whether it's an illness, the loss of a loved one, or something else, is an opportunity. It's our responsibility to discover what that opportunity is and how we can grow from it. So, when a circumstance arises that needs healing, it's there as an opportunity for you, and it's your responsibility to discover what that opportunity is and how to grow and change as a result. Recognizing personal responsibility is the first step to healing whatever imbalance it has caused.

Intention, the Master Tool

Your mind, emotions, thoughts, actions, and beliefs are all powerful influences in your physical and etheric health. The intention to heal and the belief that healing is possible are the main reasons that placebos—inert substances such as sugar pills—are so effective in clinical trials. One meta-analysis showed that patients respond positively to placebos about 35 percent of the time. Belief in a sugar pill is powerful enough to bring about change, so imagine how powerful you can be when you intentionally set out to heal.

I believe all healing is self-healing, and all self-healing starts with the intention to change. Intention is directed energy. It's more than a goal; it's a driving principle that's the foundation on which all energy healing is built. Your intention is your placebo; only it's even stronger than a sugar pill. Your intention directs your focus and energy to facilitate balance of body, mind, and spirit.

Meditation

Meditation is an excellent way to focus your intention and get into a positive and peaceful state. For our purposes, meditation is any activity you use to quiet and focus your mind. It involves being present and gently letting go of thoughts that arise, particularly negative or self-limiting beliefs.

Meditation is also an essential tool for energy healing because it creates the healing mindset you need in order to heal. I see meditation as a reset button that clears negative programming and lets you set your intention. Meditation allows you to "float away" into etheric realms where energy healing occurs, and it provides the opportunity to visualize what your experience will be and how it will feel when you are free from whatever issue you are trying to address.

Meditation gives you the tools you need not only to believe you can heal but also to allow yourself to experience and practice the sensation of healing so you can bring it into your daily life. After each meditation, you use grounding techniques to anchor the experience in your body and on the planet to manifest your healing intention in the physical realm.

MANTRAS IN MEDITATION

Many people use mantras in meditation. Traditional mantras are of Hindu and Buddhist origins, and they were originally a single word or phrase in Sanskrit, such as om (the sound of the universe) or om mani padme hum (which means "the jewel in the lotus"), that focused the mind during meditation and kept other thoughts at bay.

Over the years, mantras have evolved beyond just spiritual phrases. You can create any mantra you wish to use during a meditation. It can be a word, such as *health* or *wellness*, or it can be a phrase, sentence, affirmation, or statement of intention, such as, "I am healed," "I am healthy," or "I give thanks that I am in optimal physical, mental, emotional, and spiritual health."

Use your mantra throughout meditation, repeating it aloud or in your mind over and over again. As thoughts arise, allow them to drift away, and return your focus to your mantra.

TYPES OF MEDITATION

Many are intimidated by the idea of meditation, believing it means sitting still in the lotus position (cross-legged with the feet on the thighs) for long periods with a completely empty mind while chanting a mantra. Back when I believed that was the only form of meditation, it sounded like torture.

Although sitting cross-legged and chanting works for many people, this technique isn't for everyone. And if meditation sounds like torture to you, you're unlikely to do it. Fortunately, there are other ways to meditate, and you can get in a position that is comfortable for you. Here are a few:

Mantra Meditation: Mantra meditation is repeating a mantra as I described earlier. Choose a mantra and use it as your point of focus, gently returning your attention to your mantra whenever you notice thoughts arising. This works well for addressing specific or general health issues.

Visualization: In a visualization meditation, you create a "movie" in your head of what your life will be like after you've achieved your intention. During this type of meditation, visualize the details of your life as if you've already achieved the healing. What do you do? What do you think? How do you feel physically and emotionally? Make this movie as real as possible. This type of meditation is ideal for helping you achieve goals and intentions.

Guided Visualization: In a guided visualization, you work from a script or recording and visualize what the script or recording tells you to. This works especially well for things like clearing energetic blockages and balancing energies.

Affirmation: In affirmation meditations, you have a list of affirmations, written as positive statements, about things you intend, such as, "My body functions exactly as it should," or "I sleep deeply, soundly, comfortably, and peacefully, and I awake refreshed each morning." You repeat these affirmations aloud or in writing, or you read them throughout the course of your meditation. Affirmations are good for helping you achieve healing goals.

Sound Meditation: With sound meditation, you focus on a sound—one you make vocally, play by striking an instrument, or listen to through headphones. Sound meditations are particularly helpful with physical issues.

Movement Meditation: This form of meditation involves movement practices, such as yoga, dance, walking, or mudras (also known as hand yoga, these are hand positions you hold to create energetic shifts). During the meditation, you keep your mind focused on the movement practice and the flow of energy it creates. If your mind wanders, you gently bring it back to the movement. This is especially good for balancing and redistributing energy. (When mudras are called for in this book, an illustration accompanies them.)

HOW TO MEDITATE

Meditating doesn't need to be difficult. It's a simple process that is meant to be pleasant.

WHERE TO MEDITATE

Choose a space that's peaceful and makes you feel happy. Go where you're unlikely to be disturbed; I have an upstairs studio where I can shut out my dogs. Make sure the space has soft lighting, as well.

WHAT YOU NEED FOR MEDITATION

What you need depends on the type of meditation you'll be doing. Find a comfortable spot, such as some cushions on the floor, a comfy chair, or even a couch or bed. You'll also need a light blanket to keep you warm, comfortable clothes, supportive footwear if you're doing walking meditation, a glass of water nearby, a timer, and anything you plan to use during your meditation, such as a singing bowl or your phone.

BEFORE YOU MEDITATE

Turn off anything that will distract you during meditation, such as push notifications, particularly if you'll be playing music on your computer, smartphone, or tablet. If possible, leave elsewhere any devices you aren't using. If there's anything that you need to do, do it before you meditate, or it will be on your mind the entire time. It's also a good plan to use the bathroom before you begin.

TO MEDITATE

Once you've eliminated as many outside distractions as possible, set a timer for the amount of time you plan to meditate. Then, get comfortable and close your eyes. Breathe deeply, in through your nose and out through your mouth, noticing as the air moves down through your lungs and into your body. If thoughts arise, acknowledge them and then gently release them. Once you're in a state of relaxation, begin whatever meditation activity you are doing.

AFTER MEDITATION

When you're done, ground your energy so you return it to your body by visualizing roots growing from your core and extending deep into the earth. When you open your eyes, take a sip of water to further ground you.

Hands-On Healing

When children hurt themselves, one of the first things they do is grab the area of the injury. Why? Even very young children instinctively know there is healing energy in the hands and human touch. That's why children feel better when their moms kiss their boo-boos. Human contact is healing because it involves an exchange of energy, and when that contact is intentionally kind and loving, it brings loving energy to both parties. Touch is a way to share energy and bear witness to another in a supportive and compassionate manner. Your own touch can serve a similar function.

HEALING OTHERS

As I mentioned before, all healing is self-healing. Even as a professional energy healer who works regularly with healing partners, I understand I am not the one responsible for their healing; they are. I am merely a conduit, and I only work with people who ask for my help. I never attempt to help others heal without their permission.

Energy healers have a strict code of ethics. Even if we have the ability to send energy healing at a distance, we never do it without specific requests and permission. Nobody has the right to impose healing on another, even if they believe it will help. The path of each individual is his or her own, and it's not up to anyone else to judge whether it needs to change.

Even with a bevy of energy healing techniques under your belt, it's important to remember you only have the ability to heal one person: yourself. It is not your responsibility, nor do you have the ability, to heal another, but everyone has the capacity to *help* others heal when assistance is requested. If someone asks you to help them heal, teach the techniques you've learned, and always remember each person's healing path is uniquely their own. It's never your call to decide someone needs healing or how that healing should occur.

SIMPLE TOUCH

Simple touch requires no instruction or attunement. It is a way to send loving energy through the warmth of the hands to the part of yourself that needs healing. Try the following techniques.

TOUCH TECHNIQUE

To perform the touch technique, simply lay your hand or hands on the area where you wish to receive the energy, for example, the heart chakra.

This allows you to transmit energy from the universe into your heart, and it allows you to pull energy from the heart and send it into the universe. In simple touch, place your hands in a way that is comfortable and comforting. If possible, warm them first by rubbing them together so your touch is pleasant. Touch helps calm and harmonize energy and direct it to various places in your body.

STROKE TECHNIQUE

A stroke is stimulating and helps awaken, strengthen, and move or direct energy. To perform this technique, stroke lightly with your palms in the direction you wish energy to move. For example, if you wish to stimulate heart energy and then move it into your throat, you can lightly stroke over your heart chakra in an upward direction, increasing the length of the stroke until you pull the energy from the heart to the throat. This technique is also good for clearing blocked areas of energy in meridians or balancing the elemental energies in your body.

TAPPING

Tapping is the method by which you can perform the Emotional Freedom Technique (EFT). Developed by Gary Craig and introduced in 1995, EFT helps balance and move energy along the meridians, so it's an effective technique to use when thoughts and beliefs that don't serve you get stuck in the body. For each tapping session, focus on one belief that doesn't serve you. Come up with the problem, and then come up with an affirmation that states that the problem is gone. For example, if your problem is anxiety, the affirmation might be, "I feel calm and peaceful," or "I release anxiety."

When you employ EFT, use your pointer and middle fingers on your dominant hand—the hand you use to write or throw a ball with—to tap firmly at least five times on the following points in order:

Side of nondominant hand: Pinkie side of the hand you'd strike with to perform a karate chop

Top of head: The center of your crown

Eyebrow: Inside each eyebrow, where your brow meets your nose

Side of eye: Outside corner of each eye

Under eye: Bone just below the center of each eye

Under nose: Space between your nose and your lip

Under lip: Indent above your chin and below your bottom lip

Collarbone: Clavicle where it meets your sternum on each side

Under arm: Just below the armpit on each side of your body

As you tap on the side of your hand, say aloud, "Even though I have (problem), I deeply and completely accept myself." Then, begin the tapping sequence, starting with the top of your head. Repeat your affirmation over and over as you tap each point.

ENERGY POINTS

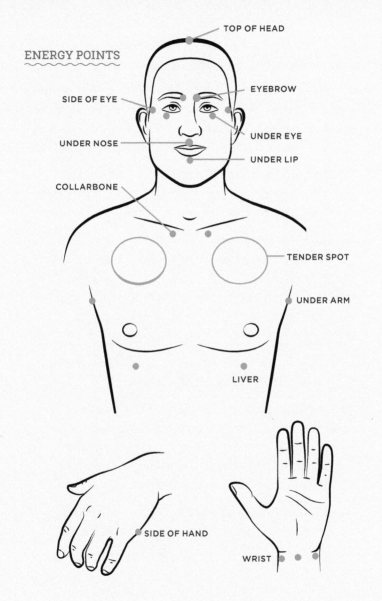

TOP OF HEAD

EYEBROW

SIDE OF EYE

UNDER EYE

UNDER NOSE

UNDER LIP

COLLARBONE

TENDER SPOT

UNDER ARM

LIVER

SIDE OF HAND

WRIST

OTHER TOUCH MODALITIES

A number of touch modalities require training or attunement. If you've already learned and are attuned to these touch modalities, feel free to use them for self-healing in the remedies and routines in place of simple touch.

Reiki is a hands-on and distance healing technique requiring training and attunement through a Reiki Master/Teacher, either in person or through a distance session.

Quantum-Touch® involves channeling energy from the earth and the universe and sending it through your hands or fingers into a healing partner or yourself. To become a Quantum-Touch practitioner, you need to attend several seminars online or in person.

Healing Touch was developed in the 1980s. To become a Healing Touch practitioner, you need to take a series of classes and workshops in the program.

Polarity therapy is a hands-on wellness practice that balances and harmonizes energy among positive and negative poles, as well as balancing the elemental energies: earth, air, fire, water, and ether. It requires multiple training courses and certification.

Acupuncture and acupressure focus on balancing energy in the meridians and clearing blockages. Training and certification are required.

Reflexology uses points in the hands and feet to free energy. Training and certification are required.

Sound Healing

If you doubt that sound affects the vibration of everything around it, try listening to live music. Notice that you feel it in your body. Music has the capacity to change your mood, affect your attitude, and more. Have you ever felt deeply moved by a piece of, say, classical music? Chances are you were reacting to the vibrational intention of the sound.

Sound's vibrational nature is demonstrated by the practice of some doctors to use a tuning fork to diagnose fractured bones. They will strike the fork and place it at the site of the suspected fracture. The vibration of the sound from the tuning fork will cause the pain in the fracture to increase.

You can bring sound into your energy healing practices in multiple ways. Some, such as using mantras and chanting, involve only your voice. Others require downloading a free or inexpensive app on your smartphone or tablet. Alternatively, you can use a crystal or bronze singing bowl during your healing practices.

BIJA MANTRAS

Bija mantras are single syllables you can chant to stimulate and activate your chakras. Each chakra has its own Bija mantra. You can use this in meditation, chanting each of the mantras in turn or focusing on a single chakra at a time and chanting the Bija mantra for that chakra over and over.

Root chakra: *Lam*, pronounced *lahm* and drawn out—*lahhhhhhhmmmmmmm*

Sacral chakra: *Vam*, pronounced *vahm* and drawn out—*vahhhhhhhmmmmmmm*

Solar plexus chakra: *Ram*, pronounced *rahm* and drawn out—*rahhhhhhmmmmmm*

Heart chakra: *Yam*, pronounced *yahm* and drawn out—*yahhhhhhhhmmmmmm*

Throat chakra: *Ham*, pronounced *hahm* and drawn out—*hahhhhhhhhmmmmmm*

Third eye chakra: *Aum* or *Om*, pronounced *ohm* and drawn out—*ohhhhhhhmmmmmmm*

Crown chakra: silence

VOWELS

If you don't want to have to remember the Bija mantras or you worry about mispronouncing them, you can also chant the vowel sounds associated with each chakra to activate and balance your chakras (see page 56). Draw the sounds out in a manner similar to that described in the previous section.

SINGING BOWLS

Singing bowls are easy to play, and I like to use them in meditations and energy healing work. There are two main types of singing bowls you can use: metal and crystal.

METAL SINGING BOWLS

These bowls are typically made from brass or bell-metal (high tin) bronze. The bronze bowls are of higher quality than the brass bowls, particularly if they are handmade in the Himalayas (you'll often see them called Tibetan singing bowls).

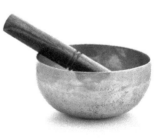

HEALING VOWELS

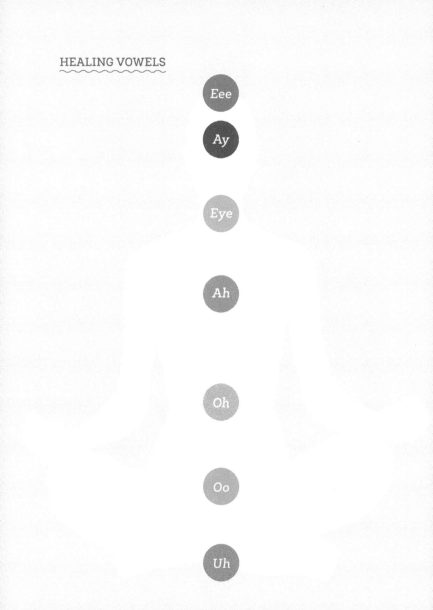

Tibetan Buddhists believe these singing bowls transmit the *dharma* (all the teachings of the Buddha) when they are played, and they emit multiple notes when you strike or ring them. They work with your body's entire energetic system rather than with a single chakra.

CRYSTAL SINGING BOWLS

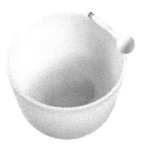

These bowls are made from crushed quartz crystal or a combination of quartz and other crystals. They play a single note when you strike them, and they tend to be tuned to a single chakra. With crystal singing bowls, the notes are as follows: C and C# for the root chakra, D and D# for the sacral chakra, E for the solar plexus chakra, F and F# for the heart chakra, G and G# for the throat chakra, A and A# for the third eye chakra, and B for the crown chakra.

APPS

Smartphone, tablet, and computer apps offer an array of sound-healing options. Here are a few:

CHAKRA TUNING

Apps such as Chakra Tuner play a series of tones that connect with each chakra. You can usually set the duration of each tone. Listen to a chakra tuning app with headphones and visualize each chakra as the tone plays. You can also set the apps to repeat one chakra if you need to balance a single chakra.

SOLFEGGIO FREQUENCIES

Solfeggio frequencies are sounds that vibrate at a certain frequency and correspond to different areas of your body. They may be specific tones or pieces of music tuned to that tone. Apps such as Solfeggio Sonic Meditations use music and sounds tuned to a certain frequency to balance or stimulate certain energies. The solfeggio frequencies are based on notes used in Gregorian chants, and each helps balance energies according to certain intentions.

396 Hz: resolving fear, safety, and guilt issues (root chakra)

417 Hz: clearing blockages or getting unstuck (sacral chakra)

528 Hz: manifesting and creating (solar plexus chakra)

639 Hz: forgiveness, compassion, relationships (heart chakra)

741 Hz: communication and creative expression (throat chakra)

852 Hz: intuition and psychic ability (third eye/ crown chakra)

963 Hz: connection to the Divine (crown chakra)

SOUND BATH

Apps such as Gong Bath allow you to relax as the vibrations of sacred healing instruments wash over you.

BINAURAL BEATS

Binaural beats are specific patterns of sound that switch between the right and left ear to stimulate different types of brain waves. You need to listen to binaural beats with headphones. Apps such as BrainWave stimulate your brain waves to reach alpha, beta, delta, or theta states to stimulate various types of healing, such as better sleep or reaching deeper meditative states.

Crystals

Crystals are rocks and minerals with a crystalline structure. There are hundreds of different types of crystals, and each has its own frequency and healing properties. You can discover more about the healing properties of crystals online or by using a good book that lists different crystals and their properties.

Each crystal vibrates at its own frequency based on its color, opacity, and internal structure. When you bring them into your environment, they entrain with the energy of beings and things near them, meeting somewhere in the middle. The result is that crystals raise the vibrational frequency of everything around them while slightly lowering their own frequency. Once they've entrained to the energy of something else, you can cleanse them to return them to their original high vibration. This causes the crystals to once again entrain and raise the frequency of what is near them to a higher level than it was before. In this way, you can use crystals over long periods of entrainment and cleansing to continuously raise the vibration of anything in their space.

Crystals are easy to use. You can bring them into your environment, and, as long as you cleanse them occasionally, they will continue to work even if you don't do anything else with them. However, when you use them with intention, they become even more powerful. Use them in other ways, by wearing them, meditating with them, making crystal elixirs (but *only* as described later in the energy healing routines), or placing them on your body during meditation or healing rituals.

An easy method to select the right crystal is to choose one with a color that matches the chakra associated with the issue you're seeking to resolve.

Red/black—root chakra: physical issues associated with the lower extremities, safety and security, depression

Brown/orange—sacral chakra: your role in your family/community, creative ideas, prosperity, sexuality, stomach, sexual organs

Yellow/gold—solar plexus chakra: self-esteem and related issues, ribs, kidneys, adrenals, liver, gallbladder

Green/pink—heart chakra: love, anger, bitterness, grief, forgiveness, heart, lungs, mid-back

Blue—throat chakra: creative expression, judgment and criticism, speaking your truth, throat, mouth, neck, thyroid

Violet/purple—third eye chakra: critical thinking, reasoning, intuition, sleep, addiction, head, eyes, ears

White/clear—crown chakra: systemic health problems, bones, skin, mental health issues, connecting to a higher power

SEVEN CRYSTALS TO OWN

The seven crystals I recommend here are affordable and easy to find, and each connects to one of the chakras, so you can use them in any of the healing rituals in later chapters. (You'll also find additional crystal choices for each chakra in the Quick Guide to Chakras and Energy Healing Tools on page 150.)

Black tourmaline: This root chakra crystal is a great all-purpose crystal. It is grounding and can block negative energy and turn negative energy into positive energy. Black tourmaline can also help with root chakra issues such as fear, safety, and security. If you can't find it, substitute **hematite.**

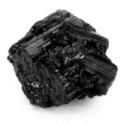

Carnelian: A form of agate, carnelian has a bright orange color, and it's plentiful and inexpensive. Use it when working with the sacral chakra to stimulate prosperity, overcome sexuality issues, or ease any struggle you may have in

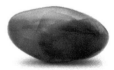

understanding where you fit in with your community or family. If you can't find it, substitute **smoky quartz.**

Citrine: Citrine is the yellow form of quartz. Lighter-yellow citrine is naturally occurring (it grows that way), whereas dark-yellow, orange-yellow, 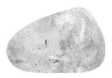 or brown-yellow citrine are all created by heat-treating smoky quartz or amethyst. Regardless of whether it's natural or heat treated, the vibrational frequency of the color will work in the same way. Citrine is naturally a prosperity stone, but it also helps with issues related to the solar plexus. It can help strengthen self-esteem and personal will as well. If you can't find citrine or it doesn't speak to you, substitute **tiger's eye.**

Rose quartz: This pretty pink stone is plentiful and afford-able. It's the naturally occurring pink version of quartz, the second-most abundant min-eral on the planet (the first is feldspar). Rose quartz is a heart 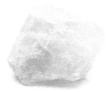 chakra stone and is great for fostering unconditional love, romantic love, forgiveness, and compassion and for releasing anger and bitterness. If you can't find it, substi-tute **moss agate.**

Celestite: Celestite has a serene blue color and pretty, sparkly crystals. It gets its blue color from the metallic element strontium. Celestite is a lovely throat chakra crystal, and it can help with communication, creative expression, and speaking your truth. It's 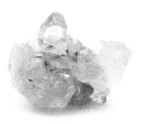 also good for thyroid or throat issues and mouth, teeth, jaw, and gum issues. If you can't find it, substitute **chalcedony** or **blue lace agate.**

Amethyst: Amethyst is the purple form of quartz. It is known as the sober stone because it's great for people in recovery. It's also a traveler's stone for safe passage. Amethyst can enhance sleep, facilitate meaningful dreams, and 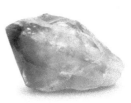 help connect you to your intuition. It supports the third eye chakra and also eases migraine headaches, mental problems, and eye problems. If you can't find it, substitute **kunzite.**

Clear quartz: You'll find clear quartz in every crystal shop you visit. It's a universal healing stone that can also amplify the power of other stones and direct their energy. In addition, clear quartz can balance the crown chakra and facilitate connection to a higher power. In the unlikely event you can't find it, try **howlite.**

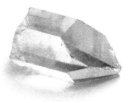

SHOPPING FOR CRYSTALS

My favorite way to purchase crystals in shops or at mineral shows is to select crystals I am drawn to. The next time you have a chance to purchase crystals in person, try this:

1. When you get to the store, sit in your car or pause outside for a moment, close your eyes, and take a deep breath, in through your nose and out through your mouth.

2. Say in your mind, "Take me to the crystals that will serve my highest and greatest good."

3. Then, when you feel calm and relaxed, enter the store. Pay attention to where you feel drawn. Move to that section of the store.

4. Once there, notice any crystals that catch your eye.

5. Pick up and hold a few crystals to see if you feel a "click" or a knowing.

6. Focus on how the crystal makes you feel and where you feel it in your body. If the crystal feels comfortable, it's the right crystal for you.

You can also purchase crystals online. There are two sites that I particularly like because the proprietors are knowledgeable and I know the quality of their crystals: BestCrystals.com and HealingCrystals.com. You can trust both of these shops to provide high-quality crystals that are advertised honestly on their websites.

PREPARING TO USE CRYSTALS

Once you get the crystals home, immediately cleanse them. You can cleanse your crystals by putting them in a singing bowl and ringing it, holding them in the smoke from a sage bundle, incense, or palo santo wood; or by leaving them in the moonlight or sunlight for 12 hours. I recommend cleansing crystals at the following times:

- As soon as you get them home from the store

- After using them in meditation or healing rituals

- When someone else has handled or used them

- After periods of discord in your home or life, such as after an illness, an upsetting life change, or an argument

- At regular intervals (a few times a week for crystals you wear and at least once a week for all your crystals)

When cleansing at regular intervals, you can simply wave the smoke of burning incense over your crystals.

Aromatherapy

Plants are living beings we share the planet with. They have very special healing properties, and aromatherapy is a great way to bring the healing energy of plants into your life. Aromatherapy uses essential oils, which are purely distilled and highly concentrated plant essences, to bring about healing.

Sacred herbs and plants have long been used in healing traditions, not just as medicines but also to change the energy of situations. They've been used by virtually every culture and form of spirituality throughout history in ritual and for medicinal purposes. For example, ancient Egyptians used plants both for religious rituals and as burial herbs to facilitate the crossing of the soul to the spiritual plane. In feng shui (the Chinese art of placement to facilitate energy flow), certain plants are used to help bring different types of energy into spaces. Native Americans burn herbs to energetically cleanse spaces. The Catholic church uses incense in its rites and rituals to carry prayer to the heavens.

Although many people understand the medical benefits of aromatherapy, they don't understand that essential oils also affect energy. Essential oils use the pure energy of plants to shift energy in the areas where they are applied or diffused. Each oil has its own vibration that can entrain to human vibration and raise it.

There are two primary ways to use aromatherapy: topically and through diffusion. With topical aromatherapy, you put a few drops of the essential oils in a carrier oil (pure vegetable or nut oils) or some other substance to dilute them, and then apply it to the exterior of the body, such as rubbing it on the skin or bathing in it. With diffusion, you put the oils in a diffuser with water, which disperses their scent into the air. You can also use a spray bottle or a diffuser for the blends I share in chapter 4.

SEVEN ESSENTIAL OILS TO OWN

There are dozens of available essential oils, and they all have their own special properties. Each of the oils noted here connects to one of the chakras, so you can use them in any of the healing rituals described in chapter 3. You'll also find more choices for each chakra in the Quick Guide to Chakras and Energy Healing Tools on page 150.

Geranium—root chakra: Grounding, safety and security, manifestation, protection, repelling negativity, balancing energies. Alternatively, try **cinnamon** or **patchouli.**

Orange—sacral chakra: Uplifts, energizes, prosperity, letting go, creative ideas, happiness and joy; helps with issues related to the sexual organs. Alternately, try **neroli** or **mandarin.**

Lemon—solar plexus chakra: Clarity, strengthens immunity, self-confidence, self-esteem, uplifts, clears blockages; helps with issues of the kidneys, bladder, gallbladder, and liver. Alternatively, try **lemongrass** or **melissa.**

Rose otto—heart chakra: Inner strength, forgiveness, love, compassion, inner peace, grief, sadness; helps with issues related to the heart and lungs. Alternatively, try **jasmine** or **vanilla.**

Roman chamomile—throat chakra: Speaking your truth, releasing judgment and criticism, confidence, acceptance; helps with issues related to the throat and sleep. If you're allergic to ragweed, don't use it. Alternatively, try **carnation** or **bay.**

Lavender—third eye chakra: Meditation, purification, spiritual growth, addiction, sleep, dreams, psychic ability and intuition, spiritual love, overcoming abandonment. This is one of the best all-purpose essential oils, so this is one you need. There are no alternatives for lavender.

Sandalwood—crown chakra: Sacred spaces, purification, connection to the Divine, meditation; helps spirits to cross over. Sandalwood is expensive, so if you need something more affordable, choose **rosewood** or **cedarwood**, which have similar properties.

SHOPPING FOR ESSENTIAL OILS

There are so many essential oil providers that it's hard to know where to look. Here are a few points to keep in mind as you shop:

- Look for oils made from organic materials.

- If the oil is packaged in plastic, steer clear. Plastic can leach into the oils, so dark-colored glass is best.

- Don't buy perfume or fragrance oil. It's synthetic fragrance that doesn't contain plant material.

- Avoid companies that charge the same price for all their oils. Essential oils vary in pricing based on the materials they contain. If they all have the same price, they're likely synthetic or made from low-quality materials.

- Check the label and make sure the oils aren't diluted. If they are, the ingredients will list some type of vegetable oil along with the plant matter.

- Beware of the words "aromatherapy grade" or "fragrance grade." These indicate an inferior product; look for therapeutic-grade products.

- You'll also need a carrier oil to dilute the essential oil. Sweet almond oil, jojoba oil, and fractionated coconut oil are all affordable, fragrance-free, healthy oils to use.

- If you're blending your own oils, you'll need small roller or dropper bottles for mixing, a dropper, and a spray bottle.

My favorite brand of essential oils is Edens Garden, although I do use oils from a few other trusted manufacturers as well. I like Edens Garden because it offers a great combination of quality, price, and variety. See the Resources section for other recommendations.

ESSENTIAL OIL PRECAUTIONS

Always dilute essential oils with a carrier oil or water before use. Although essential oils and water will not mix, water can dilute oil with the help of an emulsifier. Never apply essential oils directly to the skin; doing so can cause a sensitization reaction, such as a severe rash or breathing difficulties. If you have a reaction, stop using the oil. If you're allergic to the plant used to make the oil, don't use it.

Because of the highly concentrated nature of the oils, you should always wear gloves when you work with them to keep them from getting directly on your skin. If you have pets, talk to your vet before diffusing essential oils because diffused oils may be toxic to small animals, especially to cats. Never use essential oils internally (don't eat or drink them) unless directed to do so by a certified professional, and then only use food-grade oils. Never place essential oils directly on or near mucous membranes, such as the eyes or in your nose.

3

Daily Energy Healing Routines

One of the easiest ways to bring the power of energy healing into your life is by adopting a daily routine. Research suggests that it takes an average of 66 days of consistent behavior to create the associations in the brain that turn routines into habits. This book offers you a choice of two daily routines. Select one on the basis of your available time and perform it each day. After 10 weeks, you will have established the habit of an energy healing practice.

Drawn from meditation practices and the toolkit in chapter 2, this chapter's daily energy healing routines are arranged according to the time it takes to complete them: one is designed to take about 5 minutes to do, and the other, about 15 minutes. No matter how busy our lives are, it's likely each of us can find 5 minutes in a given day for an energy healing routine. I recommend that everyone start with the 5-minute routine to get comfortable with it and to internalize the steps to the point at which they become natural. I've included the 15-minute routine, which builds on the core steps of the 5-minute routine, for those who are able to carve out more time and experience the deep peace associated with longer energy healing rituals.

You can perform the routine of your choosing in conjunction with meditation, by itself, or even in lieu of meditation. I like to meditate for about 20 minutes before performing a ritual. Keep in mind that you can also work any of the other energy healing practices in chapter 4 into your ritual.

It's best to try to perform your healing ritual at the same time each day, but I understand this isn't always possible. I perform my rituals twice a day: first thing in the morning and right before I go to sleep. However, there are times when I have to adapt throughout the day. When this happens, I always try to find a time to squeeze it in. What's important is bringing the rituals into your life consistently and intentionally.

Before You Begin

Before you begin your daily ritual, you'll need to do some quick, basic prep work to come up with an intention. Then, you'll perform the ritual with that intention in mind.

1. Make a list of the things you'd like to heal in your life. Go ahead and make this list as comprehensive as you wish.

2. Now, narrow it down to one or two things that are the most important. These will be the first issues you work on, but keep the list of the others as well. I keep mine in a journal, and when I feel ready to move on to another, I return to my journal and find which issue feels intuitively right to work on next.

3. For each issue, create a new page. As you'll only be focusing on one or two issues right now, you'll need only a page or two for this.

4. Write the issue as a single word at the top of each page. So, you might write something like "prosperity" or "thyroid."

5. Under that, write two to three bullet points describing what your life will look like when that issue is healed. Write them as easy-to-remember affirmations. For example, for prosperity, you might write, "I have all

the money I need to be happy, healthy, and success-ful," or, "I give thanks that money flows to me easily whenever I need it."

6. Now, write a bulleted list of emotions you will feel when your problem is resolved. For example, you might feel happy, relieved, free, joyful, and so on.

CREATE AN ANCHOR

In each ritual, you'll also use a technique from the behavior-modification system known as neuro-linguistic programming (NLP). NLP was originally developed by Richard Bandler and John Grinder. The NLP technique you'll use in this book, called *anchoring*, will allow you to return to the positive state achieved in your meditation as you go about your day. With anchoring, you create positive feelings through the visualizations in your daily rituals, which are based on the affirmations and emotions you just created.

To do this, once you are in this highly positive state at the end of your ritual, make a unique gesture (such as placing your left hand over your heart or squeezing your fist tightly) and hold it until the positive feelings begin to dissipate. Then, release the gesture. This sets the ges-ture as an anchor that allows you to recall the positive feelings throughout the day when negativity arises, and it interrupts negative thought patterns that are counter-productive to healing. For example, as an anchor, I use the "okay" gesture by touching the tip of my thumb to the tip of my index finger. Come up with a gesture of your own that is easy to make but one you don't normally perform. This will anchor that feeling to the gesture. Always hold it until the blissful feelings start to fade.

As you go through your day, pay attention to your thoughts. When thoughts arise that are related to the issue you're trying to heal, make the gesture to bring back the positive feelings from your visualization and reset your intention for healing. This interrupts the energy of the negative thought. For example, if your issue is prosperity and you notice the thought arising, "I can't afford that," or a worry such as, "How am I going to pay for X?" make your gesture. You can even repeat one of your affirmations as you do, such as, "I give thanks I am prosperous." Do this every time you notice these negative thoughts arising.

RITUAL SETUP

Your setup for your ritual can be as simple or as complex as you like. As with meditation, it's important to find a place to complete your ritual where you won't be disturbed by pets, people, or electronics. If you have a space where you meditate, this is a great place to perform your ritual.

If you don't have a lot of room, even a bedroom with the door closed will work. Just let others in your household know that, during these times, you wish to be left undisturbed. As I mentioned, you can perform the ritual as an add-on to your meditation, use it in lieu of meditation, or do it separately from your meditation. It's up to you. Adapt your ritual to your own personal needs and schedule.

Some things I like in my space when I perform healing rituals for myself include the following:

- Soft music, white noise, or binaural beats

- Crystals

- A timer (this isn't necessary, but if you have limited time, it can be helpful)

- Pleasant aromas from candles, incense, aromatherapy, or herbs

- Anything in use during the ritual, such as particular crystals, a singing bowl, or essential oils

You may find something else you like. Taking the time to set up your space serves as a trigger to get you in the mind space to perform your ritual. It's a form of preconditioning so that when you begin, your mind is already primed to move to a space of positivity and healing.

My pre-ritual routine takes less than five minutes.

1. I set up cushions in my meditation space and adjust the lighting so it is soft. Normally I do this with an ambient light, such as a Himalayan salt lamp, and turn off overhead lights.

2. I light a piece of palo santo wood or nag champa incense and walk the perimeter of the room with it, waving the smoke into the corners. Then, I place the incense in a burner or the palo santo wood on a plate and let it smoke. I put the burner or plate somewhere near me where I won't accidentally knock it over or step on it. I allow the smoke to burn out on its own during my ritual.

3. If I won't be using a sound-healing instrument during my ritual, I use an app called Brainwave Studio, which uses music or ambient noise (such as birds singing or wind chimes) and isochronic tones (similar to binaural beats, but you don't need headphones) to create brain-wave states for meditation or relaxation. My apps are on my smartphone, so I also disable my ring or put my phone on "do not disturb" so I won't be distracted during my ritual.

After the Ritual

After your ritual, take a quick moment to ground yourself and return to your physically centered self. You can do this in any of the following ways:

- Visualize roots growing out from the bottom of your feet and into the earth.

- Hold a piece of black tourmaline for a moment or two in your receiving (nondominant) hand.

- Touch the ground with both hands.

- Drink a glass of cold water.

- Run your hands and wrists under cold water.

5-MINUTE DAILY HEALING RITUAL

The following ritual takes about five minutes to complete. If you wish, you can place a crystal that corresponds with the color of each chakra (see the Crystals section in chapter 2, page 60) on or near each of your chakras.

Before you begin, take a quick look at the pages where you wrote the one or two issues you'll be working with today, reminding yourself of the affirmations and emotions. Keep the pages nearby for reference if you need them during your ritual.

1. Breathe and center.

Sit or lie quietly and comfortably with your eyes closed. Take a deep breath, in through your nose and out through your mouth, allowing any tension in your body to drain from you into the earth. Allow the earth to absorb and neutralize the tension. Take three to four slow breaths.

Now, place your hands on your heart. Notice the warmth of your hands sending energy to your heart center.

Become heart centered. To do this, think of someone you love deeply or think of something for which you are profoundly grateful. Notice the love building in your heart. Spend about one minute doing this.

2. Visualize love and energy.

Visualize that love expanding from your heart and into the rest of your body, pumping through your blood vessels with every beat of your heart. Feel it expanding into every area of your body and out beyond your body into your energy field. Take about one minute to do this.

As the energy permeates you, visualize your root chakra, noticing where it touches the earth. See it as a glowing red wheel of light. You can chant the Bija mantra or healing vowel for that chakra (see the Bija Mantras section in chapter 2, page 54).

3. Move the energy.

Move the energy upward through each chakra, beginning with the root chakra. Chant the Bija mantra or healing vowel for each chakra as you visualize the movement of the energy. Visualize the sacral chakra as an orange wheel of light, the solar plexus chakra as a yellow wheel of light, the heart chakra as a green wheel of light, the throat chakra as a blue wheel of light, the third eye chakra as a violet wheel of light, and the crown chakra as pure white light. Moving the energy through the chakras should take about one minute.

4. Affirm and visualize healing.

Turn to your issues. Repeat your affirmations for each issue and then visualize yourself with those issues resolved, making this look and feel as real as possible. Allow yourself to feel the emotions you've indicated you'll feel, because your issue has been resolved. Do this for about a minute and half to two minutes.

5. Anchor and return to your body.

Now, with all of these wonderful feelings running through your body, create your anchor gesture and hold it until the positive feelings begin to subside.

When you're ready, stop the gesture and come back into your body. Open your eyes and go about your day.

15-MINUTE DAILY HEALING RITUAL

The following ritual takes about 15 minutes to complete. If you wish, you can place a crystal that corresponds with the color of each chakra (see the Crystals section in chapter 2, page 60) on or near each of your chakras.

Before you begin, take a quick look at the pages where you wrote the one or two issues you'll be working with today, reminding yourself of the affirmations and emotions. Keep the pages nearby for reference if you need them during your ritual.

1. **Breathe and center.**

   Sit or lie quietly and comfortably with your eyes closed. Take a deep breath, in through your nose and out through your mouth, allowing any tension in your body to drain from you into the earth. Allow the earth to absorb and neutralize the tension. Take three to four slow breaths.

   Now, place your hands on your heart. Notice the warmth of your hands sending energy to your heart center.

   Become heart centered. To do this, think of someone you love deeply or something for which you are profoundly grateful. Notice the love building in your heart. Spend about one minute doing this.

2. Visualize love.

Visualize that love expanding from your heart and into the rest of your body, pumping through your blood vessels with every beat of your heart. Feel it expand into every area of your body and out beyond your body into your energy field. Take about one minute to do this.

3. Visualize light energy.

With your receiving (nondominant) hand remaining on your heart center, move your giving (dominant) hand to your root chakra.

Visualize the energy running from your heart as a white or golden light, moving through your hand, down your arm and through your body, and into the root chakra.

Notice the white or golden light from your heart merging with the red light of your root chakra.

Working at about one minute per chakra, move your giving hand to each chakra, visualizing the white loving light from your heart chakra moving into each chakra and blending with the colored light there. (See page 61 for a description of the light colors associated with each chakra.) Work from root to crown. As you send the light to each chakra, you can chant the Bija mantras or healing vowel sounds associated with the chakras (see the Bijas Mantras section in chapter 2, page 54).

4. Focus on your issues.

Bring to mind the one or two issues you are working on today. Working one at a time, focus fully on these issues, noticing where you feel them in your body. See them as shadows in your body, dark smudges that are blocking the light and energy.

5. Visualize light healing.

Notice the shadows and place your giving (dominant) hand over them, with your receiving (nondominant) hand still on your heart center. Visualize the white or golden light flowing from your heart into your receiving hand, up your arm and through your body, and into your giving hand and then from your giving hand into the shadow.

Visualize this light first surrounding the shadow and then permeating it, starting to break it up into tiny pieces that blend with the light.

Visualize the pieces of blended light and shadows flowing out of your body and into the earth, where the earth absorbs and neutralizes them.

Now, visualize the once-shadowy space filled with golden or white light.

For five minutes (longer if needed), send the golden or white healing light to every issue and every shadow and watch them disappear into the earth, where they are neutralized by the earth's energy.

6. **Center, anchor, and return to your body.**

Return to your heart center. Once again, feel the light from your heart center flowing through you until you feel peaceful, relaxed, positive, and free.

Now, with all of these positive feelings running through your body, create your anchor gesture and hold it until the positive feelings begin to subside.

When you're ready, stop the gesture and come back into your body. Open your eyes and go about your day.

4

Healing Issues with Energy Work

For more condition-specific energy healing, you can pick and choose from the remedies in this chapter or use them in conjunction with your daily routine for general healing. What matters is establishing a daily practice with the intention to heal and a focus on rebalancing your energy system through the use of the various energy healing tools and techniques. Consistency and intention are far more important than the activities in which you engage, although the condition-specific practices that follow provide a framework for focusing your intention as you embark upon your healing journey.

Step into Healing

Chapter 3 offers a sequence of energy healing modalities to rebalance your energy. But you don't need to follow this sequence. Select one or more remedies suggested by your Divine guidance. There's no right or wrong way to incorporate these remedies into your self-care.

The one thing that is necessary when you work on these remedies is your intention to heal. I say it a lot, but I'll say it again: Intention is everything. Without intention, no healing tool will be effective; so with every remedy you try, it's important to maintain your focus on your intention. Although the daily routines in chapter 3 are designed to help you establish and maintain this focus on intention, the remedies in this chapter target energy imbalances that often cause specific conditions.

One way to bring your intention to the forefront as you use these tools is to state your intention aloud or silently as an affirmation before you start, and then perform the anchor gesture you created in your daily routine to bring yourself to a positive and focused state of intent. Then, allow your awareness and Divine guidance to draw you to the healing ritual you need right now. If you find another way that helps you focus on your intention, use that instead. There's no right way to do this—just options.

ABANDONMENT, FEAR OF

TECHNIQUES: AROMATHERAPY, CRYSTALS, SIMPLE TOUCH, TAPPING, VISUALIZATION

Fear of abandonment arises from wounds we experienced early in life, such as poor attachment to our parents and loss of loved ones or friends. This fear is one of the most common issues that continues to affect us as adults, causing energy imbalance and dis-ease.

Black Tourmaline and Carnelian Healing Touch

Fear of abandonment arises from feeling unsafe (root chakra) and attachments to family, friends, or community (sacral chakra). Therefore, crystals that support these areas can help. Do the following for 5 to 10 minutes:

1. Go to a place where you won't be disturbed. Sit comfortably.

2. Hold freshly cleansed black tourmaline in your receiving (nondominant) hand and place that hand over your root chakra. Hold freshly cleansed carnelian in your giving (dominant) hand and place that hand over your sacral chakra.

3. Visualize fear flowing out of your root chakra and being absorbed by the tourmaline. Visualize healing orange light flowing from your hand through the carnelian and into your sacral chakra.

Essential Oil Epsom Salt Bath

Epsom salt removes negative energy by absorbing it. The essential oils support your root and sacral chakras, which are often imbalanced when you fear abandonment.

¼ cup Epsom salt

10 drops geranium essential oil

10 drops orange essential oil

> Run the bath and add the Epsom salt and essential oils under the running water. Relax in the bath for about 10 minutes, breathing in the aroma. Before you step out and dry off, allow the water to drain completely from the tub, visualizing your fear of abandonment going down the drain.

Tapping for Abandonment

Use the tapping sequence on page 50. As you tap, repeat the following:

> Side of hand: "Even though I fear abandonment, I love and accept myself completely."

> Remaining points: "I am safe. I am loved. I am never alone."

ACUTE PAIN

TECHNIQUES: CRYSTALS, SIMPLE TOUCH, VISUALIZATION

Acute pain typically lasts fewer than six months, but it serves as an alarm to let you know something is unbalanced. It arises from recent damage or disharmony. Although most people believe pain is purely a physical sensation, it can also be etheric. Therefore, you can use these remedies for deep spiritual, emotional, or mental pain, as well as physical.

Black Tourmaline Pain Absorption

In a location where you won't be disturbed, place freshly cleansed black tourmaline on your area of pain. Lie quietly for 10 minutes. Visualize the crystal drawing out the pain energy. Do this for up to 10 minutes every hour until your pain lessens or goes away.

Laser Beam Technique

Hold the tips of your thumb, forefinger, and middle finger together on your giving (dominant) hand to create a directed beam of energy. Next, stroke this beam over an area of pain, either a few inches above the area if the pain is sensitive to the touch or severe, or right on the area if touch doesn't contribute to the pain. Repeat every hour until the pain goes away or repeat if it resurfaces.

Receiving Hand

Hold your receiving (nondominant) hand above or directly on the area of the pain. For one to two minutes, visualize your hand drawing the pain into it. Touch your hand to the ground to discharge the pain into the earth and neutralize it.

Giving Hand with Clear Quartz

Place a piece of freshly cleansed clear quartz on the area of pain. Place your giving (dominant) hand lightly on top of it. For one to two minutes, visualize healing energy flowing from your hand through the quartz and into your pain. See the pain breaking up with the energy.

Visualization

Sit or lie comfortably in a place where you won't be disturbed. For two to three minutes, visualize your pain as heat. Now, visualize cool, blue energy flowing into your pain. See the pain breaking up with the energy and dissipating up through your skin and into the universe. Repeat every hour until the pain goes away or repeat if it resurfaces.

ANXIETY AND WORRY

TECHNIQUES: AROMATHERAPY, CRYSTALS, SOUND HEALING, TAPPING, VISUALIZATION

My dad used to tell me that 95 percent of the things I worried about last year didn't happen. He was right. Worrying is never productive. It saps life force with looping thoughts that keep you in a permanent state of fight or flight, causing imbalances that can lead to dis-ease.

Lavender and Amethyst Bath

Lavender and amethyst are both soothing and calming.

¼ cup Epsom salt (optional)

10 drops lavender essential oil

1 to 2 pieces freshly cleansed amethyst

1. Run the bath and add the Epsom salt (if using) and essential oil under the running water.

2. Place the amethyst in the tub, away from where you'll be sitting.

3. Relax in the bath for about 10 minutes, deeply breathing in the aroma. If worries arise, release them and return your focus to the lavender and amethyst.

Root Chakra Sound Healing

Anxiety arises from fears about safety and security, which are root chakra issues.

1. Lie back comfortably in a location where you won't be disturbed.

2. With headphones on, listen to the 396 Hz solfeggio frequency for about 10 minutes.

3. As you listen, visualize white healing energy running through the red energy center of your root chakra.

Tapping for Anxiety

Use the tapping sequence on page 50. As you tap, repeat the following:

Side of hand: "Even though I am worried about (fill in the blank), I completely accept and deeply love myself."

Remaining points: "I feel deep peace and acceptance, and I trust the universe is conspiring in my favor."

ATTACHMENTS AND SURRENDER

TECHNIQUES: AROMATHERAPY, CRYSTALS, MEDITATION, VISUALIZATION

We sometimes attach to things that don't serve our highest good. For example, we might attach to items we no longer need or outcomes we think we want but aren't the best for us. When you recognize attachment to something that doesn't serve your highest good, use energy healing techniques to release it.

Mantra Meditation and Visualization

1. Go where you won't be disturbed, such as your meditation spot.

2. Meditate for 10 minutes, repeating the mantra, "I release (fill in the blank)."

3. As you repeat the mantra, visualize what you need to release flowing from your body and into the earth.

Rose Quartz Elixir with Rose Otto Essential Oil

Rose quartz helps you let go with love, so it's great for things like grudges or anger. Rose otto has a similar vibration and also helps with love and forgiveness. Keep in mind that quartz-based crystals are nontoxic as long as they are cleansed; but, as a general rule, when making elixirs, do not *put the crystals in the water or allow the water to come into contact with the crystals because some crystals will release toxic elements into the water.*

1. Place a freshly cleansed piece of rose quartz in a small, clean, sealed jar.

2. Pour 1 cup of water into a bowl and place the sealed jar inside. Leave it in overnight.

3. Remove the jar from the bowl and set it aside. Pour the water from the bowl into a bottle and add 10 drops of rose otto essential oil and ½ teaspoon of Himalayan pink salt.

4. Each night before you go to sleep, visualize what you need to release. Then, shake the bottle well, wet your hands with a few drops of the elixir, and smooth it over your face as you say, "I release (fill in the blank)."

Ksepana Mudra Meditation

The ksepana mudra is a simple position involving both hands that facilitates letting go of attachments that don't serve you.

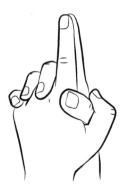

1. Hold your hands (as indicated) at the level of your heart chakra.

2. Inhale and turn your wrists so your index fingers point away from you and toward the floor. Exhale and sweep your arms over your head, extending them completely and pointing your index fingers at the ceiling.

3. Inhale and bring your hands down in front of your third eye, fingertips up. Exhale and return your hands, still holding the mudra, to the level of your heart chakra.

4. Repeat for eight cycles.

AUTOIMMUNE DISORDERS

TECHNIQUES: AFFIRMATIONS, CRYSTALS, VISUALIZATION

Around 23 million Americans suffer from one of 80 to 100 different types of autoimmune diseases. In energy healing for autoimmune diseases, you'll need to focus on three things: the root and crown chakras and the chakra closest to where the condition affects you. For example, I have Hashimoto's thyroiditis, which is related to my throat chakra. Someone with type 1 diabetes would focus on the solar plexus region, and someone with a systemic condition (such as a skin condition, rheumatoid arthritis, or lupus) would focus on the crown and third eye chakras.

Immune-Strengthening Affirmation

During your daily meditation, repeat this simple affirmation for five minutes: "I am vibrantly healthy and happy, and my immune system functions perfectly."

~~~~~~~~~

Tourmaline, Quartz, and Chakra Crystal Elixir

For this elixir, use a piece of freshly cleansed black tourmaline, clear quartz, and the crystal for the chakra closest to your most prevalent symptom. For example, if you have Grave's disease, a thyroid disorder, use a blue stone such as celestite. When making elixirs, be mindful not to put the crystals in the water or allow the water to come into contact with them because some crystals will release toxic elements into the water.

1. Place the freshly cleansed crystals in a small, clean, sealed jar.

2. Pour 1 cup of water into a bowl and place the sealed jar inside. Leave it in for 24 hours.

3. Remove the jar from the bowl and set it aside. Pour the water from the bowl into a bottle.

> Bath: Add 2 tablespoons of the elixir to your bathwater along with ¼ cup of Epsom salt and 10 drops of lavender essential oil. Soak for 10 to 15 minutes each day.

> Self-care: Add 5 drops of the elixir to your beauty products, such as your lotion or shampoo.

Chakra Clearing for Immune Balance

Gather the seven crystals or their substitutions recom-mended in chapter 2 on page 62 and go to a quiet place where you won't be disturbed. Then do the following:

1. Lie comfortably. Place your freshly cleansed crystals on the area of each chakra as follows:

> BLACK TOURMALINE—ROOT CHAKRA
>
> CARNELIAN—SACRAL CHAKRA
>
> CITRINE—SOLAR PLEXUS CHAKRA
>
> ROSE QUARTZ—HEART CHAKRA
>
> CELESTITE—THROAT CHAKRA
>
> AMETHYST—THIRD EYE CHAKRA
>
> CLEAR QUARTZ—CROWN CHAKRA

2. Breathe deeply, in through your nose and out through your mouth.

3. Visualize energy coming through the clear quartz into your crown chakra. Now visualize the energy traveling from crystal to crystal through each of your chakras, feeling the energy of the crystals balancing each chakra as it moves through.

CONTINUED

4. Once you've reached your root chakra, visualize the energy running up and down through the chakras from crystal to crystal and moving freely. While doing so, repeat the mantra, "My immune system is healthy, balanced, and strong." When you're ready, open your eyes.

"I Am the Light" Meditation

This meditation, which takes about 15 minutes, is designed to help bring energy and light to every area of your body, which can be extremely helpful with autoimmune conditions. You can use this transcript or listen to it in on my website. (See the Resources section, page 164.)

1. Sit or lie comfortably. Close your eyes and breathe deeply, in through your nose and out through your mouth.

2. As you focus on your breathing, notice that the air you are breathing is light. Visualize breathing golden or white light deeply, in through your nose and out through your mouth.

3. As you breathe in the light, see it traveling through your nasal passages and into your lungs, filling your lungs and chest with light.

4. Now, move your focus to your crown chakra, just above the top of your head. Notice your crown chakra open, and feel white light pouring in through your crown chakra, swirling down through your third eye chakra, and filling your entire head. If you were to open your eyes or mouth right now, light would stream from them and fill the space around you. Visualize looking at and listening to the world through your new eyes and ears of light, and notice how everything you see and hear is light forming the sights, colors, shapes, and sounds you recognize in your everyday life.

5. See yourself opening your mouth and light streaming out. Know that as you speak, everything you say is of the light and filled with light. Everything you place in your mouth—everything you drink, chew, and swallow— is light that nourishes and fills your entire body.

6. As the light fills and streams from your head in all directions, notice that now it is flowing downward, filling your throat and passing easily through your throat chakra. Light fills your vocal chords and carries on your voice as you speak, as you sing, as you sigh.

CONTINUED

7. The light continues downward now, traveling into your shoulders. Notice the light stream down both arms, through your elbows, into your forearms, then into your hand and fingers. The light streams from your hands and fingers. With every movement of your upper extremities, you emit light; it flows gracefully and easily, filling the space around you. As you lift your hands, as you touch objects around you, not only are you emitting light, but everything you touch, everything you feel, and everything you tap or stroke is light, as well.

8. Return your attention to your shoulders and notice the light stream down through your shoulders into your chest and upper back. The light flows into your heart and fills it. Now, as your heart beats, it pushes the light through every blood vessel in your body. The light is circulating through your veins now.

9. Notice as the light moves downward from your heart, flowing easily through your heart chakra and into your rib cage, down through your solar plexus chakra and into your abdomen. It fills your abdominal cavity, moving easily through your solar plexus chakra and through your sacral chakra, filling your entire torso and expanding down to and through your root chakra.

10. Notice the light move into your buttocks, hips, and thighs now, moving easily down through your knees, into your lower legs, ankles, feet, and toes. It streams from the bottom of your feet into the earth and out from your toes into the universe. Every cell of your body is light now; it gives light and receives light.

11. Become aware of your environment: the sounds, the smells, the feel of whatever you are sitting or lying on. Notice that these, too, are light. As you move, you are light, moving through light, breathing light, touching light, being light.

12. When you are ready, return your attention to your breathing. Notice that as you breathe in and out, the light flows freely to you, from you, and through you. When you are ready, open your eyes and walk in the world as light.

BAD HABITS

TECHNIQUES: AFFIRMATIONS, CRYSTALS, SOUND HEALING, TAPPING

Habits form as a result of repetition, eventually becoming unconscious behaviors we often don't notice we're doing. Bad habits are behaviors and choices that no longer serve our greatest good, and they often become addictions. Breaking them requires intentional effort.

Amethyst and Release Mantra

Amethyst is known as the "sober stone" because it helps remove addictions and addictive behaviors. When working with bad habits, cleanse your amethyst daily.

Each day, carry the amethyst with you in a pocket or wear it. When you recognize you're engaging in the bad habit, hold the amethyst in your receiving (nondominant) hand and repeat the mantra, "I release (fill in the habit) because it no longer serves me."

Sacral Chakra Stimulation

Bad habits often result from stuck energy in the sacral chakra, so stimulating this area regularly can help move the stuck energy.

1. Go where you won't be disturbed, and lie back comfortably.

2. Place freshly cleansed carnelian on your sacral chakra.

3. Chant the Bija mantra *Vam* or the healing vowel sound *ooo* to stimulate the chakra. As you chant, visualize energy flowing freely through your sacral chakra. Continue for two to three minutes.

Tapping to Break Habits

Use the tapping sequence on page 50. As you tap, repeat the following:

Side of hand: "Even though I have (fill in the blank) habit, I deeply and completely accept myself."

Remaining points: "I release (fill in the blank) habit because it no longer serves me."

CHRONIC PAIN

Many conditions, such as autoimmune disorders and old injuries, can leave you feeling mild, moderate, or severe pain that lasts beyond a few days or weeks until it becomes chronic. Chronic pain can be the cause of ongoing stress; it's extremely difficult to wake up and live every day in pain. Energy healing techniques can help you manage this pain.

Amethyst Point Meditation

Amethyst is a well-known cure for pain. Using double-terminated amethyst points helps direct healing energy. You'll need at least two freshly cleansed amethyst points to do this; more are better.

Place amethyst points around areas of pain with the narrow points pointing at the pain and the wide part of the point facing outward to gather energy from the universe. Larger areas will require larger points. Lie back and close your eyes for five minutes. Visualize energy flowing from the point into the pain and dissolving it.

Chronic Pain Aromatherapy Blend

Some essential oils have been shown to help relieve chronic and acute pain. Rosehip oil and Saint-John's-wort oil are especially good for relieving pain and inflammation, whereas sandalwood and lavender soothe and release heat. This blend makes 30 mL (1 ounce). NOTE: Saint-John's-wort oil is not an essential oil, but it is especially good for nerve pain. If you're struggling with things like sciatica or neuropathy, try to find it. When I buy it for my blends, I purchase it on the Internet because it isn't available locally.

1 tablespoon rosehip essential oil
1 tablespoon Saint-John's-wort oil (optional; see note)
5 drops sandalwood essential oil
4 drops lavender essential oil

Add all of the ingredients to a dark-glass dropper bottle and shake to mix well.

Bath: Add 20 drops to a warm Epsom salt bath and soak for 15 minutes.

Massage: Massage ¼ teaspoon on areas of pain, such as into the stomach for menstrual cramps or IBS pain or into the temples for migraine pain.

CHRONIC PAIN

Amethyst Roller

Place some freshly cleansed amethyst chips inside an aromatherapy roller bottle. Fill the bottle with the Chronic Pain Aromatherapy Blend on page 109. Allow it to infuse overnight. Roll it onto areas of pain as needed. (You can purchase an amethyst roller ball for the bottle in place of the chips, if you'd like.)

Baltic Amber Jewelry

Baltic amber is fossilized tree resin, so it isn't technically a crystal; but it does have anti-inflammatory effects and other healing properties that can help relieve pain.

Wear Baltic amber jewelry at the location closest to the pain. For example, for carpal tunnel syndrome, wear a Baltic amber bracelet or ring. For headaches, choose a Baltic amber necklace or earrings. For lower body pain, carry Baltic amber in your pants pocket or wear a Baltic amber anklet.

Binaural Beats

I used to have chronic migraines for more than 15 days out of the month, which took a huge chunk out of my life. Then I discovered the power of sound healing. I used binaural beats specifically for my headache pain, and it worked better than most medications. This is good for all types of pain. On iOS devices, try the app Pain Killer 2.0; on Android devices, try the app Pain Relief 2.0.

1. Go someplace quiet and dark, where you can get comfortable and won't be disturbed. Optimally, you can lie down, but sitting in a quiet room is fine, too. If comfortable, consider laying your head down on a desk or table.

2. Put on your headphones and close your eyes. Relax, and run the program for 5 to 10 minutes or until you notice the pain subsiding.

Balance Pain Meditation

Chronic pain is a message to you from your body about your physical, mental, emotional, or spiritual condition. If you ignore it, you can't heed its messages. This meditation allows you to listen to your pain and hear what it is trying to tell you. You can use this in conjunction with any of the pain techniques. This meditation calls for an anchor gesture at the end (see the Create an Anchor section in chapter 3, page 76), so create one you aren't already using, before you begin. This meditation takes 5 to 10 minutes.

1. Sit or lie quietly where you won't be disturbed. Place both hands at or near the area where you feel pain, if you can do so comfortably.

2. Close your eyes and breathe deeply, in through your nose and out through your mouth. Do this until you feel yourself relaxing.

3. Now, bring your attention to your pain. Feel it in your body, allowing yourself to experience it fully.

4. Feel the warmth from your hands flowing into your pain and loosening it.

5. Next, notice the space around your pain. Can you feel where the pain begins and ends? Notice just how much space there is not only around your pain but also between the points where you have pain.

6. Shift your focus between noticing your pain and noticing the spaces around it where the pain doesn't exist. Do this for a few minutes until you begin to notice yourself detaching from your pain.

7. In your mind's eye, as you focus on your pain, say, "Tell me what I need to know." Spend a few minutes focused on your pain and notice any thoughts or feelings that arise as you do.

8. When a thought or feeling arises, think, "Thank you," and say, "I release you." Visualize your thought or feeling dissipating into the space around you along with your pain.

9. If your pain has lessened or dissipated, make your anchor gesture and hold it for a minute or two.

10. When you're ready, open your eyes.

11. If you notice your pain starting to flare up throughout the day, make your anchor gesture.

COMPASSION

Compassion originates in the heart chakra. Therefore, working with remedies for this chakra can help you find compassion for yourself or others.

Rose Quartz and Rose Otto Heart Oil

Rose quartz and rose otto oil share a similar vibration: that of compassion and love. Together, they create a powerful remedy to help you experience deeper compassion for yourself and others. This blend makes 30 mL (1 ounce).

Freshly cleaned rose quartz chips

1 ounce carrier oil

20 drops rose otto essential oil

Place a few pieces of rose quartz chips in the bottom of a clean dropper bottle. Add the carrier oil and essential oil. Mix well. Massage ¼ teaspoon into your heart chakra in a clockwise direction three times per day.

Shuni Mudra for Compassion

Go to a location where you won't be disturbed, and get in a comfortable position. Place each of your hands in the shuni mudra, a mudra for patience, by touching the tip of your thumb to the tip of your middle finger on each hand to make a circle and rest your hands in your lap with your palms facing up.

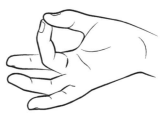

As you hold the position, focus on your heart chakra and repeat, "Compassion" for five minutes.

Heart Chakra Solfeggio Frequency

Lie back comfortably in a place where you won't be disturbed, and with headphones on, listen to the 639 Hz solfeggio frequency for about 10 minutes. As you do so, visualize your heart chakra opening and pouring love and compassion into the universe.

ENERGY BALANCE

Balancing energy involves balancing polar energies, creating balance among the elemental energies, and allowing a free flow of energy through your chakras. Each of the techniques here outlines a way to balance one of these types of energies.

Metta Sutta Yin Yang Balance Sound Meditation

For this technique, you will strike your singing bowl or sound the tone on a singing bowl app as you recite the Metta Sutta, a Buddhist discourse on loving-kindness, line by line. Allow the bowl or tone to ring until the sound completely decays before you strike it again. Strike it and state as follows:

Strike 1: "May all beings be peaceful."

Strike 2: "May all beings be happy."

Strike 3: "May all beings be well."

Strike 4: "May all beings be safe."

Strike 5: "May all beings be free from suffering."

Elemental Energy Balancing

For this technique, use a freshly cleansed clear quartz crystal—preferably a point. Refer to the illustrations in the Meridians section of chapter 1 on page 30 to see how to visualize each energy channel. Plan to spend about five minutes on this visualization.

Place the tip of the crystal on the big toe on your right foot and visualize the energy running up the channel in the diagram, clearing it. Continue in this order for each energy as follows: right big toe, left big toe, right second toe, left second toe, right middle toe, left middle toe, right fourth toe, left fourth toe, right pinkie toe, left pinkie toe.

Chakra Balancing

For this technique, you will need to gather the seven crystals (or their substitutions) recommended in chapter 2 on page 62.

1. Go to a quiet place where you won't be disturbed, and lie comfortably.

2. Place your crystals on the area of each chakra as follows:

   BLACK TOURMALINE—ROOT CHAKRA

   CARNELIAN—SACRAL CHAKRA

   CITRINE-SOLAR PLEXUS CHAKRA

   ROSE QUARTZ—HEART CHAKRA

   CELESTITE—THROAT CHAKRA

   AMETHYST—THIRD EYE CHAKRA

   CLEAR QUARTZ—CROWN CHAKRA

3. Chant the Bija mantra or healing vowel sound for each chakra as you visualize energy moving through the root chakra to the crown chakra and back again. When ready, open your eyes.

FORGIVENESS

Forgiveness is a huge issue for so many. When we hold on to the energy of pain that we believe another has caused us, it doesn't hurt the other person; it hurts us. This is because it continues to generate negative energy from the precipitating event long after it transpired. When we forgive, we refuse to allow negative energy from the past to affect us now.

Forgiveness Visualization

You can perform this forgiveness visualization as part of your meditation or on its own. You only need a few minutes alone in a place where you won't be disturbed.

1. Close your eyes and place both hands over your heart chakra, breathing deeply.

2. Visualize the person you need to forgive. See the ties of hurt or anger as strands of energy connecting you to each other.

3. Now visualize a pair of scissors cutting each of the strands. As you cut the strands, say, "I release you." When the strands have all been cut, visualize each of you surrounded by a green, healing light.

CONTINUED

4. Use an anchor gesture (see the Create an Anchor section of chapter 3, page 76) to hold on to this feeling of forgiveness. Open your eyes when you're ready. If you notice your anger arising throughout the day, use your anchor and say, "Release," aloud or in your mind's eye.

Tapping to Forgive
Use the tapping sequence on page 50. As you tap, repeat the following:

> Side of hand: "Even though I am (angry/upset/hurt) about (event/person), I completely love and accept myself."

> Remaining points: "I release (name). I forgive (name)."

Rose Quartz Forgiveness Visualization
1. Sit comfortably with your eyes closed, holding freshly cleansed rose quartz in your giving (dominant) hand.

2. Imagine someone you love deeply or something that makes you feel deeply grateful and happy. When you feel the love building in your heart, visualize it moving through your arm, into your giving hand, and into the piece of rose quartz.

3. Transfer the rose quartz to your receiving (nondominant) hand. Feel the energy from the quartz flowing up your arm and into your heart as you visualize the person you need to forgive. Visualize that person moving into your heart center along with the energy of the rose quartz. As you do this, say aloud or silently, "I forgive you. I release you."

4. Hold that person in your loving energy for as long as you feel it is appropriate. Open your eyes when you're ready.

Singing Bowl Forgiveness Ritual

For this ritual, use a crystal singing bowl tuned to F or F# or a bronze singing bowl, which plays harmonics and overtones that work with all of the chakras. Alternatively, you can use a tuning fork tuned to F or F#. Plan to do this for about five minutes.

1. Sit comfortably with the bowl in front of you. Strike the bowl and let it ring. Close your eyes and breathe in through your nose and out through your mouth, allowing the sound of the singing bowl to fade naturally.

CONTINUED

2. After the sound fades, strike the bowl again. Visualize the energy of the bowl coming in through your nose and traveling down through your breathing passages and into your heart. Allow the tone to fade naturally.

3. Visualize the person you need to forgive as you strike the bowl again. Breathe in the sound as you visualize the person, bringing both your visualization and the sound of the bowl into your heart center. Allow the tone to fade naturally, still holding the person in your heart.

4. Strike the bowl and say silently or aloud, "I forgive you. I release you." Repeat this mantra as the sound fades.

5. Strike the bowl again, and, as the sound fades, visualize the hurt and anger that tied you to the other person dissolving.

6. Release the image of the other person and strike the bowl one final time. Breathe in the tone and allow it to fill you completely. When you're ready, open your eyes.

GRATITUDE

TECHNIQUES: CRYSTALS, MEDITATION, VISUALIZATION

Practicing gratitude is a foundational technique in energy healing because it helps move you into a state of positive emotions, where you can start to create healing. Cultivating gratitude is a daily practice you can use throughout the day to increase positive emotions.

Solar Plexus-Heart-Throat Gratitude Energy

Practice moving gratitude energy through the chakras. Gratitude arises in your solar plexus chakra as a function of self-worth, moves into your heart chakra to gather love, and then moves into your throat chakra, where you express it. Take as long as you need for this exercise.

1. In a place where you will not be disturbed, sit or lie comfortably.

2. Visualize something you're grateful for as you focus on your solar plexus. See it as golden energy. See the golden energy move into your heart, where it mixes with green love energy. See the golden energy move into your throat and mix with the blue energy there.

3. When you're ready, say, "I'm grateful for . . ." and express your gratitude. Repeat the cycle for each person, experience, or thing you are grateful for.

GRATITUDE

Bedtime Gratitude

As you drift off to sleep, meditate on all that you are grateful for. To do this, cycle through the alphabet in your mind. For each letter, list something in your life you're grateful for that starts with that letter. You'll likely fall asleep in the process, but it allows you to head into sleep in a positive space.

Gratitude Elixir

Citrine, rose quartz, and celestite support your middle three chakras: solar plexus, heart, and throat, which are all associated with finding, feeling, and expressing gratitude. Be mindful that quartz-based crystals are nontoxic as long as they are cleansed; but, as a general rule, when making elixirs, do not *put the crystals in the water or allow the water to come into contact with them because some crystals will release toxic elements into the water.*

1. Place a freshly cleansed piece of citrine, rose quartz, and celestite in a small, clean, sealed jar.

2. Pour 1 cup of water into a bowl and place the sealed jar inside. Leave it in overnight.

3. Remove the jar from the bowl and set it aside. Retain the water from the bowl.

Bath: Run a bath and pour the contents of the bowl into your bathwater. Bathe for 10 minutes while reflecting on the things in your life that you are grateful for.

GRIEF

TECHNIQUES: AFFIRMATIONS, AROMATHERAPY, MEDITATION

Everyone experiences grief differently, and it's important to allow the process of grief to move through you in its own way, in its own time. It's unhealthy to suppress grief. Use energy healing techniques to help you process grief in a healthy way to keep yourself from getting stuck in it.

Essential Oil Grief Blend

Essential oils such as orange and lemon are uplifting. When grief threatens to overwhelm you, use these oils in the bath or with a simple massage. This blend makes 30 mL (1 ounce).

1 ounce sweet almond oil or other neutral carrier oil
9 drops orange essential oil
9 drops lemon essential oil

Add all of the ingredients to a dark-glass dropper bottle and shake it to mix well.

Bath: Add 10 drops to a warm bath and soak for 10 minutes.

Massage: Massage ¼ teaspoon into your heart chakra.

Heart and Root Chakra Meditation

Getting stuck in grief usually happens in the energy of the root chakra, which is where we hold our sense of safety and security, or in the heart chakra, where we hold not only love and forgiveness but also anger and other intense emotional pain. You can perform this heart and root chakra meditation with crystals (rose quartz on the heart and black tourmaline at the root chakra), if you'd like. Plan for about five minutes.

1. Lie comfortably with your eyes closed. If you're using crystals, place black tourmaline on your root chakra and rose quartz on your heart chakra.

2. Allow yourself to notice any feelings of grief that arise, but try not to judge them. Instead, notice them and where in your body you feel them.

3. Bring that feeling into your heart chakra if it isn't already there.

4. Visualize energy coming up from the earth through your root chakra, and draw it up into your heart chakra to mix with your grief.

CONTINUED

5. Visualize the grief energy moving back down from your heart to your root chakra and draining from your root chakra into the earth. Feel how the earth absorbs the energy while supporting you completely.

6. Now, feel white light energy coming down from above and filling your heart. Pull that energy down into your root chakra and back up to your heart. Circulate the energy for as long as you need. When you're ready, open your eyes.

Grief Release Affirmation

Grief gets stuck when you attempt to suppress it, and it doesn't come neatly in the moments when you're alone and safe. It can come up anytime and anyplace. It's one of those situations where the only way around it is through it. You can use an affirmation to facilitate this process, once you get to a safe space where you can allow the experience.

1. Choose an affirmation that reminds you to allow the full experience of your grief instead of suppressing it. It can be something like, "Allow," or something more complex, such as, "My grief flows through me freely."

2. Anytime your grief starts to arise, take a few deep breaths. If you just can't flow with the grief in the moment, as soon as possible try to get to a place where you feel safe to experience and express your grief. It's okay to wait until you are in a place where you feel safe.

3. Now, allow your grief to arise, stating your mantra as you allow the experience to fully move through you.

4. Breathe deeply. Notice the feelings, but don't judge them. Continue repeating your mantra, allowing yourself the space to process your grief for as long as you need.

5. As your grief begins to pass, take a few deep breaths and center yourself in your heart.

6. Express gratitude for your grief. When you're ready, open your eyes.

HEALTH

Frequently, physical health issues are the first signs you recognize when energetic imbalances and dis-ease arise. They usually begin as a mild symptom, but as the imbalance magnifies, the symptoms become stronger and more persistent. Attending to your physical health, however, involves more than treating physical symptoms. The remedies in this section look beyond the physical to help remove the causes of the imbalance.

Sit with Symptoms

Sitting with symptoms allows you to hear what your body is trying to tell you.

Sit or lie quietly and comfortably, and ask yourself, "What is it I need to know?" For the next 10 minutes, quietly observe and see what arises in your body, mind, or spirit. For example, as you focus on your symptoms, anger at someone may arise. When something such as an emotion or fear comes up as you sit with symptoms, this is often the root cause. Noticing this will help you identify what is unbalanced and causing your symptoms or dis-ease, which allows you to do something about it.

Clear Quartz Health Elixir

Clear quartz is a universal crystal that helps with every issue. Be mindful that quartz-based crystals are nontoxic as long as they are cleansed; but, as a general rule, when making elixirs, do not *put the crystals in the water or allow the water to come into contact with them because some crystals will release toxic elements into the water.*

1. Place a freshly cleansed clear quartz crystal in a small, clean, sealed jar.

2. Pour 1 cup of water into a bowl and place the sealed jar inside. Leave it in for 48 hours.

3. Remove the jar from the bowl and set it aside. Pour the water from the bowl into a bottle.

> Drink: Add 1 tablespoon of the elixir to your morning water, juice, or smoothie.

~~~

Full-Body Sound Healing

This remedy is simple and quick and uses the healing vowel sounds associated with the chakras (see the Vowels section of chapter 2 on page 55 and the Healing Vowels chart on page 56). You don't need to know particular notes; you'll just slide up and down in pitch as you vocalize the vowel sounds. This practice should take just a few minutes.

1. Do the following in a single breath: Start with the root chakra vowel sound, vocalizing it in the lowest tone your voice can manage. Moving to the next chakra and vowel sound, vocalize the sound in a slightly higher tone. Do this for each chakra up to your crown chakra, vocalizing the vowels in ascending tones. The crown chakra should be the highest tone your voice can manage.

2. Breathe, and then in a single breath, head back down in pitch, vocalizing the vowels in descending tones until you return to the root chakra.

3. Perform a total of eight ascents and eight descents.

INNER PEACE

TECHNIQUES: AROMATHERAPY, CRYSTALS, MEDITATION, SOUND HEALING

World peace starts with inner peace, one person at a time. Finding and remaining in a state of inner peace is a choice that helps create the conditions ideal for healing.

Singing Bowl Peace Meditation

Sit comfortably with a singing bowl in front of you. Strike the singing bowl and let it ring. As you strike the bowl, say aloud, "My body is at perfect peace. I feel deep peace at the sound of the bowl." Allow the tone to decay completely. Strike again and repeat the phrase. Do this nine times.

Celestite Focal Point Meditation

The color of celestite is a peaceful blue that sparks feelings of serenity.

Meditate with celestite as a focal object—that is, gaze at it softly—for 5 to 10 minutes.

INNER PEACE

Peace Spray

The essential oils in this spray blend evoke feelings of peace. You can spritz your pillow with this spray before sleep or your meditation space to set the mood. This blend makes 44 mL (1½ ounces).

4 ounces distilled or spring water

1 tablespoon rubbing alcohol or vodka

1 tablespoon Himalayan pink salt or sea salt

20 drops lavender essential oil

20 drops Roman chamomile essential oil

10 drops sandalwood essential oil

Add all of the ingredients to a spray bottle and shake it gently. Spritz an area once or twice, away from your face.

JOY AND POSITIVITY

TECHNIQUES: AFFIRMATIONS, AROMATHERAPY, MEDITATION

Cultivating joy and other positive feelings is essential to energy healing. The more positive emotions, like joy, you can create in your life, the more easily you can step into the space where healing is possible.

Inner Smile Mudra (Hansi Mudra)
The inner smile, or laughter, mudra, hansi, evokes joy and positivity.

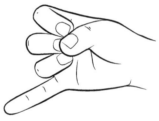

Place the tip of your thumb against the tip of your middle finger to create a circle, and then hold your ring and forefingers in the circle as well, next to your middle finger, as the image shows. Extend your pinkie out straight with your palm facing upward.

Sit and hold the hansi mudra, with both hands resting in your lap, palms facing up. For 5 to 10 minutes, repeat the affirmation, "I am filled with joy and laughter."

Joyful Massage Blend

Lemon and orange essential oils are uplifting, making for an excellent massage blend when you want to feel more joy. This blend makes 30 mL (1 ounce).

1 ounce carrier oil, such as sweet almond oil
10 drops lemon essential oil
5 drops orange essential oil

> Add all of the ingredients to a dark-glass dropper bottle and shake it to mix well. Massage ¼ teaspoon into your solar plexus chakra.

Laughter Meditation

I engage in a movement practice called Nia. In Nia, we have a practice that involves sitting and fake laughing for 30 to 60 seconds. Whenever I do it, I notice that the fake laughter quickly becomes real, and I feel real joy. This exercise may feel uncomfortable at first, but eventually the laughter will turn to real joy.

> In a place where you won't be disturbed, sit comfortably on the floor. Take a breath and begin to laugh, faking it at first. Continue to laugh for 30 to 60 seconds. Notice whether you begin to laugh for real.

LOVE AND RELATIONSHIPS

TECHNIQUES: AFFIRMATIONS, AROMATHERAPY, VISUALIZATION

It's natural to want love and companionship in your life. Loving others and feeling loved helps us create and hold positive emotions and experiences, whereas feeling a lack of love can lead to imbalance or dis-ease.

Love Magnet Visualization

Sit or lie comfortably with your eyes closed. Visualize your heart glowing with a deep green color that surrounds you with green light. Now, visualize that green light as a magnet, attracting all types of love toward you. Do this for 5 to 10 minutes.

Rose Otto and Sandalwood Love Blend

Strongly associated with your heart chakra, rose otto and sandalwood essential oils both have a vibration that supports and attracts love. This blend makes 30 mL (1 ounce).

1 ounce carrier oil, such as sweet almond oil

6 drops rose otto essential oil

6 drops sandalwood essential oil

Add all of the ingredients to a dark-glass dropper bottle and shake it to mix well. Massage ¼ teaspoon into your heart chakra.

Love Affirmation

1. On a piece of paper, write down all of the qualities you want in a love relationship, along with how such a relationship will feel.

2. Use the qualities and feelings you identified to create five affirmations, written as positive statements or statements of gratitude about a love relationship. For example, "I am grateful I have the perfect partner in my life to bring me joy," or "My life is filled with love, laughter, and friends."

3. Repeat your affirmations five times each morning when you wake and each night before you go to sleep. Continue this process for as long as you feel the need.

PROSPERITY AND ABUNDANCE

TECHNIQUES: AFFIRMATIONS, CRYSTALS, VISUALIZATION

Prosperity is a big issue for many, and our unconscious beliefs about the availability of abundance in the universe can create imbalances in our lives. Use energy healing techniques to uncover subconscious beliefs about lack and to rebalance the energy of abundance in your life.

Citrine Feng Shui for Prosperity

Citrine is the crystal most commonly associated with prosperity and abundance. You can use the feng shui sector of prosperity in your home. In traditional feng shui, it is the southeast sector or corner of your home or room. In Western feng shui, it is the back-left corner of your home or room, from the door, facing in.

Place a freshly cleansed citrine crystal in one of these sectors and carry a small piece of citrine in your wallet or purse to boost prosperity and abundance.

Abundance Visualization

Go to a place where you won't be disturbed. Sit or lie comfortably and close your eyes. Visualize yourself as a giant magnet with money flowing to you from multiple channels. As you do, repeat the affirmation, "Abundance flows to me freely from all channels." Do this for 5 to 10 minutes.

Prosperity Mindfulness

One of the keys to overcoming poverty consciousness is to practice prosperity mindfulness throughout the day. Become aware of how you think about money, as well as how often and how frequently those thoughts are of lack. For instance, if a bill comes in and you think, "I can't pay for this," you are engaging in poverty consciousness.

Create an affirmation such as, "I give thanks I have all the money I need to pay my bills and live a comfortable, prosperous life." Every time you catch yourself engaging in poverty consciousness, repeat your affirmation.

SELF-LOVE

TECHNIQUES: AFFIRMATIONS, CRYSTALS, MEDITATION, VISUALIZATION

All love and healing begin with self-love. Ironically, we often find it easy to love others and difficult to love ourselves. Finding self-love means accepting all aspects of ourselves, even those things we wish to disown about ourselves. Energy work can help you find self-acceptance for all aspects of yourself, even those aspects you wish to keep in the shadows.

Solar Plexus and Heart Elixir

Rose quartz and carnelian, as well as rose otto, orange, and sandalwood essential oils, can all enhance the vibration of self-love. Be mindful that quartz-based crystals are non-toxic as long as they are cleansed; but, as a general rule, when making elixirs, do not *put the crystals in the water or allow the water to come into contact with them because some crystals will release toxic elements into the water.*

1. Place a freshly cleansed rose quartz and carnelian in a small, clean, sealed jar.

2. Pour 1 cup of water into a bowl and place the sealed jar inside. Leave it in for 48 hours.

CONTINUED

3. Remove the jar and set it aside. Pour the water into a jar and add 20 drops of rose otto essential oil, 20 drops of orange essential oil, and 5 drops of sandalwood essential oil.

> Meditation or Bath: Transfer the contents of the jar to a spray bottle and use it to mist your meditation space before you meditate, or add 2 tablespoons to your bathwater.

Vajrapradama Mudra Meditation

The vajrapradama mudra, also called thunderbolt, is a mudra of deep self-love.

Interlace the fingertips of both hands as the image shows to make a V with both hands with the thumbs pointing upward. Hold your hands over your heart.

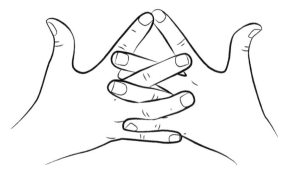

Using the image of a thunderbolt as a reference, hold the mudra over your heart as you focus on your heart chakra and repeat the affirmation, "I deeply and completely love myself." Do this for 5 to 10 minutes.

Shadow Integration Visualization

It's important to integrate the parts of ourselves that we have disowned. This simple meditation can help you reintegrate your shadows into your conscious self.

1. Sit or lie comfortably in a place where you won't be disturbed for 5 to 10 minutes.

2. Focus for a moment on all of the things you dislike about yourself. See them as shadows that form in your body.

3. Now visualize love from your heart chakra as a green light radiating from your heart center and flowing in, around, and through the shadows, causing them to break up. See the bits of the shadows mingled with green light flowing back into your heart, where they turn to love.

SPIRITUAL GROWTH

Our entire existence as spirits embodied as humans is to grow spiritually while living in a human body. This mission carries on when we are no longer embodied and exist only in spirit form. Therefore, spiritual growth is more essential to our beings than air is to our bodies.

Anjali Mudra Meditation

Also known as prayer hands or prayer position, the anjali mudra is used in yoga poses such as the tree pose and sun salutation. You don't need to be a yogi to practice anjali. Just sit comfortably with your hands in prayer position.

1. Start with your hands in front of your heart chakra. As you hold your hands here, breathe in deeply. As you exhale, think or say aloud, "Spirit, enter my heart."

2. Raise your prayer hands until they are level with your third eye. Breathe in and then out. As you exhale, repeat, "Spirit, flow through my mind."

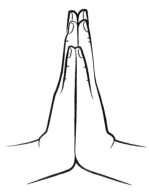

3. Move your hands, still in the anjali mudra, to above your head. Breathe in and then out. As you exhale, repeat, "Spirit, flow from above and around me to fill me with the energy of the Divine."

4. Repeat seven times.

Sandalwood and Lavender Massage Blend

This blend can help open your eyes to what you need to grow spiritually. It makes 15 mL (½ ounce).

1 tablespoon carrier oil, such as sweet almond oil
2 drops sandalwood essential oil
2 drops lavender essential oil

1. Add all of the ingredients to a dark-glass dropper bottle and shake it to mix well.

2. Place two or three drops of the blend on your fingertips. Sit comfortably with your eyes closed.

3. Massage the blend into your third eye chakra in a clockwise rotation as you say, "Spirit, show me what I need to know to grow." Repeat nine times.

4. Massage the blend in a counterclockwise motion as you say, "Spirit, help me manifest my new knowledge in my life." Repeat nine times.

Dream Meditation

This meditation is a powerful way to help you have meaningful dreams.

Place a piece of freshly cleansed amethyst, which supports dreaming, on your bedside table, on the floor beneath the head of your bed, or between the head of your mattress and box spring. Before you drift off to sleep, say, "Spirit, tell me what I need to know in my dreams."

As soon as you wake up, record what you remember from your dreams in a journal and see what you can glean from them by using a dream dictionary, such as DreamMoods.com, to interpret the symbols.

TRUST

TECHNIQUES: **AFFIRMATIONS, CRYSTALS, MEDITATION, TAPPING**

Trust issues originate in your root chakra, whereas trust-worthiness comes from your throat chakra, which is all about speaking your truth. You need to weigh the ability to trust others with your own trustworthiness to create harmony and balance.

Black Tourmaline and Celestite Meditation

Using a mantra meditation with crystals connects your root chakra (security) to your throat chakra (trust and truth), helping you learn to trust.

1. Go someplace that's comfortable and quiet, where you won't be disturbed.

2. Lie on your back with freshly cleansed black tour-maline on your root chakra and celestite on your throat chakra.

3. Visualize energy flowing from your root chakra up to your throat chakra and back down again as you repeat the affirmation, "I trust the universe, and I, in turn, am trustworthy." Do this for about five minutes.

TRUST

Tapping for Trust

Use the tapping sequence on page 50 if you have trust issues with a specific person. As you tap, repeat the following:

Side of hand: "Even though I don't trust (person) (or person doesn't trust me), I completely and fully love and accept myself."

Remaining points: "I work to safely build trust with (person). Even if (person) is untrustworthy, I am safe."

Universal Trust Affirmation

Repeat the following affirmations five times each morning and five times before going to sleep. Daily repetition will help set these affirmations as reality the more you work with and repeat them.

"I trust that the universe sends me what I need for my greatest good."

"I trust that my thoughts, words, and actions always serve my highest good."

"I trust that others do the best they can for their own good with the tools they have."

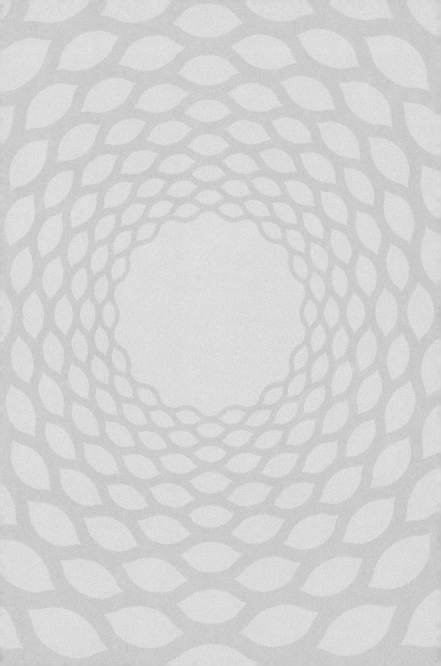

Root Chakra
(Base or Muladhara)

COLOR: RED

MANTRA: *LAM*

NOTE: C OR C#

SOLFEGGIO FREQUENCY: 396 HZ

EMOTIONAL/SPIRITUAL ASPECTS

- Abandonment
- Connection
- Grounding
- Loyalty and trust
- Oneness/ we are all one
- Place in family/ community
- Safety
- Security and protection
- Standing up for oneself
- Truth

PHYSICAL AREAS/ISSUES

- Addiction
- Bowels
- Depression
- Hemorrhoids
- Immune system
- Legs, feet,
  ankles, knees
- Lower back pain
- Rectal issues
- Sciatica
- Tailbone
- Varicose veins

CRYSTALS
Red or black crystals/magnetic crystals

- Black tourmaline
- Garnet
- Hematite
- Jet
- Lodestone
- Obsidian
- Ruby

ESSENTIAL OILS

- Cinnamon
- Geranium
- Ginger
- Myrrh
- Nutmeg
- Patchouli
- Vetiver

Sacral Chakra
(Spleen or Svadisthana)

COLOR: ORANGE

MANTRA: *VAM*

NOTE: D OR D#

SOLFEGGIO FREQUENCY: 417 HZ

EMOTIONAL/SPIRITUAL ASPECTS

- Control
- Creativity
- Finances/prosperity
- Personal power
- Relationships
- Sexuality

PHYSICAL AREAS/ISSUES

- Addiction
- Appendix
- Bladder
- Constipation/ diarrhea
- Hips
- Intestines
- Pelvic region
- Sexual dysfunction
- Sexual organs

CRYSTALS
Orange or brown crystals

- Amber
- Carnelian
- Citrine
- Copper

- Orange aventurine
- Orange calcite
- Peach moonstone
- Smoky quartz

ESSENTIAL OILS

- Bergamot
- Cedarwood
- Clary sage
- Geranium

- Orange
- Sandalwood
- Tangerine
- Ylang-ylang

Solar Plexus Chakra

(Navel or Manipura)

COLOR: YELLOW/GOLD

MANTRA: *RAM*

NOTE: E

SOLFEGGIO FREQUENCY: 528 HZ

EMOTIONAL/SPIRITUAL ASPECTS

- Belonging
- Boundaries
- Community/ group honor
- Group function
- Group safety/security
- Law and order
- Personality
- Self-esteem
- Sense of self separate from others
- Social rules

PHYSICAL AREAS/ISSUES

- Abdominal organs
- Acid reflux
- Adrenals
- Diabetes
- Eating disorders
- Gallbladder
- Kidneys
- Liver
- Mid-back
- Rib cage
- Spleen
- Stomach
- Ulcers
- Xyphoid process

CRYSTALS
Yellow or gold crystals

- Amber
- Bismuth
- Citrine
- Gold
- Heliotrope
- Pyrite
- Yellow tiger's eye

ESSENTIAL OILS

- Frankincense
- Lemon
- Lemongrass
- Roman chamomile
- Tea tree

Heart Chakra
(Anahata)

COLOR: GREEN

MANTRA: *YAM*

NOTE: F OR F#

SOLFEGGIO FREQUENCY: 639 HZ

EMOTIONAL/SPIRITUAL ASPECTS

- Anger
- Balance
- Bitterness
- Bridge between physical and etheric
- Fear of loneliness
- Forgiveness
- Grief
- Health
- Love
- Self-centeredness
- Strength

PHYSICAL AREAS/ISSUES

- Blood vessels
- Breast issues
- Breathing
- Circulation
- Heart
- Lungs
- Mid-back
- Rib cage
- Shoulders/ arms/hands
- Sternum
- Thymus gland

CRYSTALS

Green or pink crystals

- Amazonite
- Aventurine
- Emerald
- Green aventurine
- Green calcite
- Green kyanite
- Green tourmaline
- Jade
- Malachite
- Moss agate
- Peridot
- Rose quartz

ESSENTIAL OILS

- Cypress
- Geranium
- Jasmine
- Lavender
- Neroli
- Rose
- Rose otto
- Ylang-ylang

Throat Chakra
(Vishuddha)

COLOR: BLUE

MANTRA: *HAM*

NOTE: G OR G#

SOLFEGGIO FREQUENCY: 741 HZ

EMOTIONAL/SPIRITUAL ASPECTS

- Creative expression
- Following your dream
- Integrity
- Self-expression
- Speaking out
- Surrender to Divine will
- Truth

PHYSICAL AREAS/ISSUES

- Ears
- Esophagus
- Gums
- Jaw
- Mouth
- Neck
- Teeth
- Throat
- Thyroid and parathyroid
- Upper chest

CRYSTALS

Blue crystals

- Angelite
- Aquamarine
- Blue kyanite
- Blue lace agate
- Blue tiger's eye
- Blue topaz
- Celestite
- Chalcedony
- Sapphire
- Turquoise

ESSENTIAL OILS

- Bay
- Chamomile
- Eucalyptus
- Fennel
- Geranium
- Ginger
- Jasmine
- Lavender
- Peppermint

Third Eye Chakra
(Pineal or Ajna)

COLOR: PURPLE/VIOLET

MANTRA: *AUM*

NOTE: A OR A#

SOLFEGGIO FREQUENCY: 852 HZ

EMOTIONAL/SPIRITUAL ASPECTS

- Critical thinking
- Emotional intelligence
- Evaluating attitudes
- Evaluating beliefs
- Intellect
- Intuition
- Learning from experience
- Mental health
- Open-mindedness
- Psychic ability
- Reasoning

PHYSICAL AREAS/ISSUES

- Brain
- Eyes
- Head
- Headaches
- Nerves
- Nightmares
- Pineal gland
- Pituitary gland
- Sinus and eye problems
- Sleep problems

CRYSTALS
Purple or violet crystals

- Amethyst
- Blue kyanite
- Chalcedony
- Charoite
- Iolite
- Kunzite
- Labradorite
- Sugilite
- Tanzanite

ESSENTIAL OILS

- Bay
- Clary sage
- Frankincense
- Juniper
- Lavender
- Myrrh
- Peppermint
- Rosemary
- Sandalwood
- Vetiver

Crown Chakra
(Sahasrara)

COLOR: WHITE OR VIOLET

MANTRA: NONE—SILENCE

NOTE: B

SOLFEGGIO FREQUENCY: 963 HZ

EMOTIONAL/SPIRITUAL ASPECTS

- Communication with higher beings
- Communication with higher self
- Compassion
- Connection to spirit
- Divinity
- Ethics and values
- Selflessness
- Spirituality
- Understanding who we are
- Universal trust
- Walking a spiritual path

PHYSICAL AREAS/ISSUES

- Bones
- Muscles
- Skin
- Systemic issues

CRYSTALS

Clear, violet, or white crystals

- Amethyst
- Apophyllite
- Clear quartz
- Goshenite
- Moonstone

- Morganite
- Petalite
- Phenacite
- Selenite

ESSENTIAL OILS

- Frankincense
- Helichrysum
- Jasmine
- Lavender
- Neroli

- Rose
- Rose otto
- Rosewood
- Sandalwood
- Vetiver

RESOURCES

Apps

BINAURAL BEATS

BrainWave 35 Binaural Series by Banzai Labs
(Apple App Store)
Brain Waves Binaural Beats by MynioTech Apps
(Google Play)

CHAKRAS

Chakra Tuner by Jonathan Goldman, Healing Sounds
(Apple App Store)
Chakra Sound by Self Healing (Google Play)

PAIN CONTROL

Pain Killer 2.0 by Brian Zeleniak (Apple App Store)
Pain Relief 2.0 by Brian Zeleniak (Google Play)

SOLFEGGIO FREQUENCIES

Solfeggio Sonic Meditations by Diviniti Publishing Ltd.
(Apple App Store)
Solfeggio Frequencies by MediApps (Google Play)

SOUND HEALING

Gong Bath, Gong Sounds with Meditation Timer for Yoga
Healing Therapy by Rehegoo (Apple App Store)
Gong Sounds by Leafgreen (Google Play)

Books

CRYSTALS

*The Crystal Alchemist: A Comprehensive Guide to
Unlocking the Transformative Power of Gems and
Stones* by Karen Frazier (Reveal Press, 2019)
*Crystals for Beginners: The Guide to Get Started with the
Healing Power of Crystals* by Karen Frazier (Althea
Press, 2017)
*Crystals for Healing: The Complete Reference Guide
with Over 200 Remedies for Mind, Heart, and Soul* by
Karen Frazier (Althea Press, 2015)

DREAM SYMBOLS

*Dark of Night in the Light of Day: The Art of
Interpreting Your Dreams* by Karen Frazier (Afterlife
Publishing, 2017)
*Llewellyn's Complete Dictionary of Dreams: Over 1,000
Dream Symbols and Their Universal Meanings* by
Michael Lennox (Llewellyn Publications, 2015)

ENERGY

The Field: The Quest for the Secret Force of the Universe
by Lynne McTaggart (Harper Perennial, 2008)

*The Law of Attraction: The Basics of the Teachings
of Abraham* by Esther and Jerry Hicks (Hay
House, 2006)

ENERGY HEALING

*Anatomy of the Spirit: The Seven Stages of Power and
Healing* by Caroline Myss (Harmony, 1996)

*Energy Medicine: Balancing Your Body's Energies for
Optimal Health, Joy, and Vitality* by Donna Eden and
David Feinstein (Jeremy P. Tarcher, 2008)

*Higher Vibes Toolbox: Vibrational Healing for an
Empowered Life* by Karen Frazier (Afterlife
Publishing, 2017)

Quantum-Touch: The Power to Heal by Richard Gordon
(North Atlantic Books, 2006)

*Reiki Healing for Beginners: The Practical Guide with
Remedies for 100+ Ailments* by Karen Frazier (Althea
Press, 2018)

You Are the Placebo: Making Your Mind Matter by Joe
Dispenza (Hay House, 2015)

MEDITATION, MINDFULNESS, AND SELF-AWARENESS

Loving What Is: Four Questions That Can Change Your Life by Byron Katie and Stephen Mitchell (Harmony, 2002)

Meditation for Fidgety Skeptics: A 10% Happier How-to Book by Dan Harris, Jeffrey Warren, and Carlye Adler (Spiegel & Grau, 2017)

The Miracle of Mindfulness: An Introduction to the Practice of Meditation by Thich Nhat Hanh (Beacon Press, 1999)

The Power of Now: A Guide to Spiritual Enlightenment by Eckhart Tolle (New World Library, 1999)

SOUND HEALING

Ancient Sounds for a New Age: An Introduction to Himalayan Sacred Sound Instruments by Diáne Mandle (Top Reads Publishing, 2018)

How to Heal with Singing Bowls: Traditional Tibetan Healing Methods by Suren Shrestha (Sentient Publications, 2018)

The Humming Effect: Sound Healing for Health and Happiness by Jonathan Goldman and Andi Goldman (Healing Arts Press, 2017)

Tibetan Sound Healing: Seven Guided Practices to Clear Obstacles, Cultivate Positive Qualities, and Uncover Your Inherent Wisdom by Tenzin Wangyal Rinpoche (Sounds True, 2011)

Documentary Films

Heal, directed and written by Kelly Noonan. Elevative
Entertainment, 2017.

The Healing Field: Exploring Energy and Consciousness,
directed by Penny Price. Penny Price Media, 2016.

The Secret, directed by Drew Heriot. TS Production
LLC, 2007.

What the Bleep Do We Know!?, directed by William
Arntz and Betsy Chasse. Gravitas Ventures, 2005.

Websites

CRYSTAL SHOPS
BestCrystals.com
HealingCrystals.com

DREAM SYMBOLS
DreamMoods.com

EFT INFORMATION
EmoFree.com
UnseenTherapist.com

ESSENTIAL OILS
doTerra.com
EdensGarden.com
MountainRoseHerbs.com

MEDITATION TRANSCRIPT
"I Am Light" Guided Meditation and Visualization, 2018,
www.authorkarenfrazier.com/blog/i-am-light-guided
-meditation-and-visualization.

SINGING BOWLS
Bodhisattva Trading Co., Inc. Tibetan Singing Bowls:
Bodhisattva-Store.com/listings/.
Crystal Tones: CrystalSingingBowls.com
iSingingBowls.com.

REFERENCES

Benson, Kia. "Essential Oils and Cats." *Pet Poison Helpline.* Accessed April 15, 2019. http://www.petpoisonhelpline.com/blog/essential-oils-cats/.

Burgin, Timothy. "History of Yoga." *Yoga Basics.* Accessed April 15, 2019. http://www.yogabasics.com/learn/history-of-yoga/.

Gupta, Usha, and Menka Verma. "Placebo in Clinical Trials." *Perspectives in Clinical Research* 4, no. 1 (January–March 2013): 49–52. doi:10.4103/2229-3485.106383.

Hanegraaff, W. J., Antoine Faivre, Roelof van den Broek, and Jean-Pierre Brach, eds. *Dictionary of Gnosis and Western Esotericism.* Boston: Brill, 2005.

HealthCMi. "Acupuncture Reduces Post-Stroke Depression, Restores Function." *Healthcare Medicine Institute News.* March 31, 2019. Accessed April 15, 2019. http://www.healthcmi.com/acupuncture-continuing-education-news.

Mandal, Ananya. "Acupuncture History." *Medical Life Sciences News.* Last modified February 26, 2019. Accessed April 15, 2019. http://www.news-medical.net/health/Acupuncture-History.aspx.

Qingyong, He, Ji Zhang, and Yuxiu Tang. "A Controlled Study on Treatment of Mental Depression by Acupuncture Plus TCM Medication." *Journal of Traditional Chinese Medicine* 27, no. 3 (September 2007): 166–69. http://www.ncbi.nlm.nih.gov/pubmed/17955648.

Ramirez, Jonatan Peña, Luis Alberto Olvera, Henk Nijmeijer, and Joaquin Alvarez. "The Sympathy of Two Pendulum Clocks: Beyond Huygens' Observations." *Scientific Reports.* March 29, 2016. Accessed April 15, 2019. doi:10.1038/srep23580.

Röschke, J., Ch. Wolf, M. J. Müller, P. Wagner, K. Mann, M. Grözinger, and S. Bech. "The Benefit from Whole Body Acupuncture in Major Depression." *Journal of Affective Disorders* 57, nos. 1–3 (January–March 2000): 73–81. doi:10.1016/S0165-0327(99)00061-0.

Sun, Zhi-Kun, Hong-Qi Yang, and Sheng-Di Chen. "Traditional Chinese Medicine: A Promising Candidate for the Treatment of Alzheimer's Disease." *Translational Neurodegeneration* 2, no. 6 (February 2013). doi:10.1186/2047-9158-2-6.

Toney, Chelsey M., Kenneth E. Games, Zachary K. Winkelmann, and Lindsey E. Eberman. "Using Tuning-Fork Tests in Diagnosing Fractures." *Journal of Athletic Training* 51, no. 6 (June 2016): 498–99. doi:10.4085/1062-6050-51.7.06.

University College London. "Science of Habits." *UCL Healthy Habits*. Accessed April 15, 2019. http://www .ucl.ac.uk/healthy-habits/science-of-habits.

Violatti, Cristian. "Upanishads." *Ancient History Encyclopedia*. May 4, 2014. Accessed April 15, 2019. http://www.ancient.eu/Upanishads/.

INDEX

F

Feng shui, 139
Fire element, 25
Forgiveness, 119–122

G

Gallbladder meridian, 31–32
Geranium essential oil, 69, 91
Giving hand, 93
Gratitude, 123–125
Grief, 126–129
Grinder, John, 76
Grounding, 80
Guided visualization, 43

H

Habits
  bad, 106–107
  building, 73–74
Hands-on healing, 46–53
Healing. *See also*
    Energy healing
  basic practices, 33–34
  definitions of, 2
  mindset, 38
  others, 47
Healing touch, 52, 90
Health, 130–132
HealthCMI, 10

Heart chakra, 14, 18–19, 156–157
  Bija mantra, 54
  crystals, 61
  essential oils, 69
  gratitude energy, 123
  grief meditation, 127–128
  self-love elixir, 141–142
  singing bowl note, 57
  solfeggio frequency, 59, 115
  vowel, 56
Heart meridian, 29–30
Huygens, Christiaan, 10

I

Imbalance, 11–13, 16
Inner peace, 133–134
Intention, 40, 88–89

J

Jesus, 4
*Journal of Affective
    Disorders*, 10
Joy, 135–136

K

Kidney meridian, 30, 32

V

Vibration, 5–8
Visualization, 43
  abundance, 139
  acute pain, 93
  forgiveness, 119–121
  love magnet, 137
  shadow integration, 143
  surrender, 96
Vowels, 55

W

Water element, 26
Western medicine, 4
Worry, 94–95

Y

Yang, 28, 31–32
Yin, 28, 29–30, 32
Yoga, 3

ACKNOWLEDGMENTS

I am incredibly grateful for the opportunity to write about and teach something I love and believe can help people grow, change, and heal. As I was telling my friend Seth Michael recently, if something I write or teach speaks to even one person, that is reason enough to have done it. And so, I'm grateful to you, my readers and students, who summon great courage to step on the path to intentional healing. It's beautiful, meaningful, powerful, difficult work, and you're all warriors in the best sense of the word. Thank you.

Thank you to my project manager and editor at Callisto, Stacy Wagner-Kinnear, the first person to trust me to write an energy healing book (*Crystals for Healing*). In doing so, you helped one of my dreams come true, and you continue to play a vital role in that.

I'm also grateful to my husband, Jim, and my sons, Tanner and Kevin, for continuing to put up with having an author in the family and all the missed meals that occur as a result. Thanks also to my mom, Brenda, who has shown me this past year, in the wake of my dad's death, what courage and grace truly look like.

I'd also like to thank my tribe. Kristen Gray and Kasci Lawrence pulled me through what was an incredibly difficult past year with the power of love, laughter, and female friendships. The members of the Vision Collective—Sharon Lewis, Tristan Luciotti, Amy Castellano, Seth Michael, Jyl Straub, Jason and Carolyn Masuoka, Mackenna Long, Kristen Gray, and Luis Navarrete—have been a joy to work and teach with, and I'm proud to be a member.

Thank you, as well, to all of my teachers—both those who meant to teach me and those who did so accidentally. One of my life's greatest blessings is that our paths crossed somewhere along the way and I've learned from you.

And finally, thanks to my dog, Monkey. She thinks she helps when I write. Who am I to argue?

ABOUT THE AUTHOR

Karen Frazier is the author
of books about metaphys-
ics, crystal healing, energy
healing, dream interpretation, and the paranormal.
As a professional writer,
she has also ghostwritten a
number of books and penned
hundreds of articles about a
variety of topics.

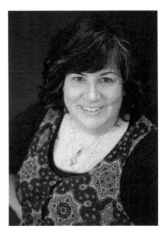

As a columnist for
Paranormal Underground
magazine, Karen cur-
rently writes two columns: "Dreams and Symbols" and
"Metaphysics and Energy Healing." She is also the
Paranormal and Horoscopes editor for LoveToKnow,
writing feng shui, numerology, palmistry, psychic
phenomena, paranormal, divination, and tarot articles
for the site. She teaches classes about energy healing,
crystal healing, sound healing, feng shui and space
energetics, I Ching and divination, dream interpretation,
Reiki, personal development, and psychic development.

Karen is an intuitive energy healer who is a Usui Reiki Ryoho Master/Teacher (Shinpiden), a Crystal Reiki Master/Teacher, a Karuna Ki Reiki Master, a Raku-kei Reiki Master, and a certified animal Usui Reiki Ryoho practitioner. In addition, Karen is an ordained minister for the International Metaphysical Ministry. She holds a bachelor of metaphysical science (BMSc) and a master of metaphysical science (MMSc) as well as a doctorate in metaphysical parapsychology. She is currently working on a doctoral thesis focusing on sound as a source of spiritual healing to earn her doctor of divinity (DD) in spiritual healing. She is also a Nia White Belt and a member of the International Association of Reiki Professionals. Likewise, Karen teaches classes at, and is a founding member of, the Vision Collective, a group of energy healers, psychic mediums, and spiritual teachers offering metaphysical courses in the Portland, Oregon, area.

Learn more at AuthorKarenFrazier.com.